Headache Solutions
at the Diamond Hea

MW00892888

By Seymour Diamond, MD
Emeritus Founder and Director, Diamond Headache Clinic;
Executive Chairman and Founder, National Headache Foundation

In collaboration with Brad Torphy, MD
Diamond Headache Clinic

With Charlie Morey
Writer, editor, graphic artist

Other books by Seymour Diamond, MD

The Headache Godfather
Skyhorse Publishing Company
By Seymour Diamond, MD with Charlie Morey

Headache and Migraine Biology and Management
Elsevier Science and Technology Books
Edited by Seymour Diamond, MD

Headache Through the Ages
Professional Communications, Inc.
By Seymour Diamond, MD with Mary Franklin

ISBN: 978-1-97993-384-1

iii

CONTENTS

INTRODUCTION

I am so happy my Dad asked me to write this introductory. It gave me the opportunity to think about what drew me into becoming a physician, and more importantly why I followed him on this great journey to help headache patients get respectful care for their chronic disease. It still surprises and emboldens me today to reach for hope for those who have none and carry them along to rejoin their lives.

My first memory of what my Dad did for a living came when I was 8 or 9 at an AMA convention in Atlantic City. My sister Judi and I were put to work manning the exhibit he had set up. His study was on the masks of depression and how tricyclic antidepressants helped people with pain. My Dad would talk to anyone who stopped, energized and passionate about his ideas.

Throughout my teenage years, people often asked what my father did. "He is a headache doctor," I would simply say. It always was met with a similar response, "Is that a thing?" Sometimes I would get embarrassed but being around my Dad I knew he was doing something special. Sadly, sometimes when I say what I do I am met with the same question, "Is that a thing?" Fortunately, today, because of the work my Dad and others I can bring so many more tools to my patients. Knowledge is power.

While growing up, we all worked at the clinic. I remember sitting with Mary Ann at the switchboard transferring calls. It was a fun plug-in one. Later I taught biofeedback with Mary Franklin. If I was being groomed for my future, I didn't know it.

Off to college at the University of Michigan, I gravitated to pre-med classes but refused to say I wanted to be a doctor. Defiant and independent, I wanted my own path, not my Dad's. I remember my senior year when he came to lecture for my sociology class on Future Worlds. He was on the class syllabus with the likes of Buckminster Fuller and Carl Sagan. I didn't realize that he was a pioneer until that day.

My parents encouraged me to apply to medical school and I did (obviously). My classmates and I worked at the clinic during our free time doing physicals. I ventured into the world of emergency medicine. I wanted to do my own thing, and I loved the adrenaline buzz. Life has a way of making us change and adapt, and I found myself craving a more normal life.

Generously, my Dad opened the door, and I joined the practice. I loved headache medicine (yes, it was a thing) and most of all I learned to be a doctor like my Dad. It's hard to describe, but he possesses the rare but amazing gift of being a wonderful clinician. He taught me to listen to the nuances, ask questions, and search for that patient what might be the best therapy. In a few words, he was the consummate clinician.

No matter where I go or who I am talking to, an amazing thing usually happens. Someone knows someone who knows my Dad. It is never unusual to have someone say, "Your Dad helped me, what a great doctor! Dr. Diamond changed my life." I smile and say right back he changed mine too!

Merle Diamond, MD

PREFACE

While browsing through some books in my medical library not too long ago, I came across an anecdote about George Bernard Shaw, the eminent British playwright and critic. It seemed both apt and incisive in terms of the subject and the attitude of this book.

Shaw, a crusty direct man, suffered from intense headaches—chronic, recurring headaches which were so devastating that he would lose a full day of work or pleasure out of every month, at least until the time he reached the age of 70.

One day, just after one of those terrible sieges of pain, he met Fridtjof Nansen, the renowned Norwegian explorer, scientist, and humanist. Nansen had explored the polar ice cap without quite reaching the North Pole and had won the Nobel Peace Prize in 1922 for his relief work in the wake of World War I.

Shaw, somewhat out of sorts from the remembered headache pain, greeted Nansen by suggesting that he had misdirected his life.

"Have you ever discovered a cure for a headache?" Shaw asked.

"No," said the somewhat astonished Nansen.

"Well, have you ever tried to *find* a cure for headache?"

"No," replied Nansen.

"Well, that is a most astonishing thing!" said Shaw. "You have spent your life trying to discover the North Pole, which nobody on earth cares tuppence about, and you have never attempted to discover a cure for the headache, which every living person is crying aloud for."

In a sense, that complaint is the starting point of this book.

We live at a time when extraordinary achievements are commonplace: we climb the highest mountain, smash the smallest atom, and reach the nearest moon. But nobody thinks much about something so commonplace and yet important as finding a way to end a pain in the head.

The headache is a universal plague. It strikes virtually everybody at some time in his or her life, even if only on rare occasions. It strikes tens of millions of Americans and hundreds of millions of people around the world as a constant, recurring, intense pain. Yet, since it has not been recognized as a universal concern, there has been no universal cure.

The fact of the matter is that headache pain is a very personal thing. It is personal in the sense of being intimate: it is both *of* the victim and *in* him. The pain seems both to possess the sufferer, while at the same time he seems to possess *it*. It is a pounding, mind-numbing, spirit-shattering pain which the victim feels not only that he cannot escape, but that nobody can help him escape. It is one thing to suffer a dreaded disease, knowing that one day there will come an end to it, either through a cure or otherwise. It is quite another thing to know that one is condemned to give up a certain number of days of one's life—and for a small number of people, *all* the days of their lives—to an agony that can neither be avoided nor escaped, that knows no cure, and that nobody but the victim takes seriously.

Headache pain is personal, also, in the sense of having a particular "fit"; that is, each victim has a kind of headache as personal to him as his hair or eye color. Since there are very many kinds of headaches, different causes, and different patterns, there can be no one cure for all headache pain. The extent to which the headache can be treated—and it can be reduced in frequency and intensity—is also an individual matter.

There is a good deal of headache research being conducted right now. A growing number of doctors are striving to learn how best to treat headache, and there is a very rewarding dialogue within the medical profession about how to attack the problem. But despite these efforts, there is noticeably little information available for the victims themselves—it seems that those most intimately concerned are the last to know what is available to ease their pain.

In this book, we are trying to share some of the facts about headaches and our understanding of them, with those more deeply affected, the headache victims. No arcane medical terms are used here. We have tried to keep the discussion deep and precise, but also conversational in tone. We are talking of individuals and their pain, not of laboratory results.

In this book, stories of mysterious and elusive headache pain are told, in many cases by the patients themselves. The author, as the doctor, intrudes to the extent of lending depth, understanding, and a certain dimension to a discussion of the problem. This is necessary because it is not only the science that we are focusing on, but how the science can be used to serve people in pain.

This book contains a total of 30 case histories and discussions of their solutions and treatments. In addition, there are appendices referencing current drugs, diets, and headache calendars. Information on current headache treatments and a dedicated hospital inpatient unit are included.

Although case histories of real people are cited, their names have been changed to protect them from any embarrassment that might occur as a result of sharing their experiences.

There are certain concepts and details of treatment that have been repeated in several chapters throughout the book. There are two reasons for this: one is to emphasize and reemphasize the kind of treatment involved in headache pain and the precautions that must be taken; the other is to make each case history as complete as possible so that the reader does not have to flip to other pages to find the reference to a treatment.

You may see familiar details in the cases related here. However, please don't jump to the conclusion that the case cited is identical to your own; that is most unlikely. Headache pain is so specifically individual to allow for easy duplication. The only safe and intelligent thing to do is to discuss with your doctor some of your insights and experiences, knowing now, after reading these accounts, what your doctor must consider to offer you the best possible treatment for your headache.

To preserve the realism of the patients' accounts of their problems, we have used trade names of drugs and the actual dosages which were prescribed.

(Each drug's trade name is indicated throughout the book within parentheses.) It should be clearly understood that all the medications mentioned in the book are to be taken only under the strict supervision of a physician, in consideration of a careful history and a diagnosis of the headache problem has been made. Dosages and types of medication will inevitably vary within each individual case.

Also, take note that you won't read the phrase "sure cure" here. There are very few certain "cures" in the treatment of headache. Medical science can be used to lessen the pain, and on rare occasions it might be ended altogether, but there is never a guarantee that it won't return or that the root cause of the headache has been eliminated forever.

What you will find here is some insight as to what is happening in this age-old, long-neglected malady; what we are trying to do in the headache field; how we are trying to do it; and how it affects the people most concerned

Seymour Diamond, MD

ACKNOWLEDGEMENTS

To Brad Torphy, MD, for his painstaking assistance in researching, writing, and editing the third edition; to William Barry Furlong, for his efforts in the original version of this book; to Elaine Diamond and Mary Franklin for their help with the manuscript; to Ira M. Turner, MD, for the chapter entitled, "Migraine Preventive Therapy: What's in the Pipeline?"; to Roger Cady, MD, and Kathleen Farmer, MD, for the appendix entitled, "Acute Medications for Migraine"; to the Academic Press for excerpts from the book *Headache and Migraine Biology and Management*, which I edited for use of charts and illustrations. Last and not least, to the actual patients who so graciously allowed their histories to be published.

Seymour Diamond, MD

To my parents, Teresa Finney and Dave Torphy, who instilled in me compassion and empathy, and to the doctors at Diamond Headache Clinic—Merle Diamond, MD, George Urban, MD, and Alex Feoktistov, MD, who afforded me the opportunity to work with headache patients and are incredible mentors to me.

Brad Torphy, MD

DEDICATIONS

To my wife Elaine of almost 70 years.

To my three accomplished daughters -- Judi, Merle, and Amy -- who tolerated their father for more than 59 years.

To my grandchildren Max Barack and his wife Debbie Simons, Michael Barack, Jacob Barack, Zachary Rose Barack, Emily Diamond-Falk and her husband Alex Horowitz, Brian Diamond-Falk and his wife Katie Steele Diamond-Falk, and three great-grandchildren Zevon, Oliver, and Veronica Diamond-Falk.

To all the patients that have passed through the doors of the Diamond Headache Clinic since 1972, and the multitude of doctors, residents, fellows, medical students, nurse practitioners, doctors' assistants, and physician assistants who have learned from their experiences with the Diamond Headache Clinic.

Seymour Diamond, MD

1

THE AD MAN'S MYSTERIOUS HEADACHE

His eyes were like caves. His face wore a vaguely haunted look.

"Good afternoon, doctor," he said as he glanced at his wrist-watch during the small formalities of greeting. "Nice office you have here."

His eyes took in the stern geometry of the examination room. My eyes followed his and took in the details: he had not moved the out-of-line chair back to the wall; he had not moved the examination gown, thrown casually onto the examination table, to line up its folds neatly with the edge of the table.

Not, possibly not, a classic migraine, I thought.

"Doctor, have you ever encountered a pain in your head so bad that you wonder if it's worthwhile going on living"? The abruptness of his question and the change of pace were typical: he seemed like a man who was already late for a plane.

"Yes," I said quietly. Hourly, I thought. To him, the pain was not only personal, it was exceptional and exclusive. But in virtually every hour of my practice at the Headache Clinic in Chicago, I encounter patients who feel the same way—desperate, driven men and women who cannot escape a headache pain so intense that they literally beat their heads against a wall to quell it or want to tear out their eyeballs to get at it. Not infrequently, as the pain goes on hour after hour, day after day, year after year, the victim wonders if this is all there is to life—if life is, indeed, worth living if all it contains is pain. "The art of life," wrote Thomas Jefferson, who was the victim of chronic, intense headaches, "is the avoiding of pain."

This patient touched the front of his head where he had the pain. Occasionally, he would brush his fingers along the side of his head where his thick, prematurely white hair was shaped ever so subtly.

"There's something very wrong up here, doctor," he said. "I feel"—his words came more hesitantly— "that it must be something serious. Like a brain tumor."

Another clue. His headaches must have come on suddenly and recently. The victims of migraine or other chronic headache problems have had them so long that they don't often worry about a brain tumor. The fact that it might be a brain tumor occurs only to those to whom the headache pain is new and terrifying.

I glanced at his chart. It had only the briefest of biographical notes. Name: Gunther Reis. Age: 51. Occupation: advertising man. He was, I would soon learn, chief executive of an account group in a very large advertising agency. He was clearly comfortable with his success and his prosperity: On this first visit, he wore a pinstriped three-piece suit, a polished cotton shirt with contrasting collar, and a polka-dot silk tie. His impatience under these circumstances was itself marked: As I would discover, his normal pace under pressure was so unhurried that he was the envy of his colleagues.

There is a great deal you can learn about a headache victim just by observing him.

- A person with a headache stemming from anxiety or depression is likely to appear quite calm and relaxed, all the while complaining bitterly of severe, disabling pain.
- A person with migraine often, not always, is high strung, likes to talk in rather quick and hurried phrases, and is extraordinarily neat and well groomed—even picky and precise. He or she is likely to be a perfectionist. That's why we leave a chair awry or an examination gown tossed carelessly on a table in the Diamond Headache Clinic. The migraine victim will, almost reflexively, line up that chair just so and fold up the examination gown, placing it on the table so that its folded edges match precisely the corner of the table.

2

- A person with a headache due to certain organic problems—something specifically wrong with an organ of the body, such as the brain—tends to walk and move quite slowly and deliberately while in pain; the jarring associated with walking often accentuates the pain.
- A person who does not swing his arms while walking may have a headache due to a certain kind of organic problem of the brain or central nervous system.
- Another patient with headaches due to certain disease of the spinal cord might walk with his feet wide apart.
- Even more specifically, a patient who had an organized problem in the outer layer of the larger part of the brain (where the supposed center of the intellect, the will, and emotions are located, and where the motor impulses originate) is likely to walk swinging a leg in a cone-like motion instead of stepping straight forward.
- A person who has trouble talking or articulating his words, and who is right-handed, may have a lesion in the left side of his or her brain.
- Indeed, you can look at the skin of some patients and get a clue to their problems: There is a reason to believe that the victims of cluster headaches, which involve very intense pain, often have thick facial skin with deep furrows in the forehead and pitted, course skin on the cheeks, somewhat like the skin of an orange.

"Suppose," I said to Gunther Reis, "you tell me how the headaches seemed to strike you."

At core, he was a plain man. His mental processes were uncomplicated. Apparently secure in his job, he seemed to possess few of the self-doubts (until the headaches struck) that affect many others in his profession. He spoke clearly and fluently of the symptoms that harassed him.

He had suffered an occasional headache throughout his life. It has been reported that 7 out of every 10 adults in America use painkillers for headaches at

3

least once a month. It is now estimated that billions of dollars are spent annually on the over-the-counter headache remedies that you see advertised endlessly on television and in other media. But the headaches that now pained Gunther Reis—the dread, piercing, pounding pain—began about three months ago. He didn't know why. It was imperative that I now do a thorough headache history. (See Appendix I, Diamond Headache Clinic Headache History.)

"Did you have an accident about that time?" Often a blow on the head, not even a terribly sharp one, will leave an injury under the outer covering of the brain that can cause headache pain. He searched his memory. He couldn't recall anything.

Was there a change in his job?

Just one: a large new account had been added to his group. But that merely increased his stature and his salary; he didn't suffer any undue pressure from the added work load. At his level, he could delegate a good deal of the added labor.

Did he have to—ah—entertain more now than in the past?

"Do you mean," he asked sharply, "am I drinking more?" He shook his head. "Less, if anything. Just a little white wine at dinner."

"How often do these headaches come?"

He thought about that. "I don't know," he said. "Irregularly, I guess." Another clue suggesting it was not migraine. Patients with migraine know precisely when and how often and how long their headaches strike. They often come in with long lists. When you have a patient with lists, you have a patient with migraine.

"How long do they last?"

"Half a day, Sometimes the better part of a day."

"Do you get any warning that they're coming on you?"

"What do you mean?"

"Well, do you 'see things'? Bright lights, maybe like the sun flashing? Or strange patterns in front of one of your eyes?"

"No. Not a thing. The headache just comes on me."

"Do you feel a little nauseated before they hit?"

"No."

"Or a little testy or irritable?"

He thought it over for a moment. "No. They just hit."

"Do you find yourself waking up very early in the morning? And then you can't go back to sleep?"

"No. I sleep pretty much as I always have. Get up about seven o'clock and get to the office about a quarter to nine."

"Do you sometimes have one of these headaches when you wake up?"

"Sometimes. Usually, though, they hit me later in the day."

"Does either of your eyes get teary or does your nose run during the headache?"

"No."

"What do you do for them?"

"I cancel all my appointments and I go home and go to bed."

This complete retreat is an important aspect of the lives of headache victims—sometimes those outside their families rarely understand. The headache pain changes, even warps, their whole way of life. It begins to interfere with the way they work and then with the way they live. A strong man or woman can literally be broken under the impact of severe, chronic, recurring headaches. Reis was aware of this. His face was showing the strain of the fight against pain.

"You take aspirin for them?"

"Lots of it."

"Anything else?"

"I can't find anything else that'll help. Even aspirin won't do it." Then, a little sheepishly, he pulled a bottle out of his pocket. "Another doctor suggested I take these."

It was sumatriptan, which was introduced in the United States in 1992. It is often very effective in treating severe migraine. (See Appendix II, Drugs Used in Acute Migraine Attacks.)

Some migraine patients get some sort of warning that the headache is starting. In migraine with aura (formerly known as classic migraine), the patient sees auras, or visions, a half-hour or so before the pain hits. He or she may also get other signals, from a feeling of nausea to a certain testiness. So the signals are there to take a triptan in time for it to be distributed by the blood system before the headache pain sweeps over the victim. Unfortunately, not all headache victims—in fact, not all migraine victims—get these signals. Many migraine victims get relief even if they take the triptan or ergotamine tartrate at the first hint of real pain. But if they don't, they can't get it into their system before the pain totally envelopes them.

"Now tell me about the pain. Where it hits. How it feels."

His response was ready enough. Pain—constant, recurring headache pain—is something the victim comes to know too well. And whether or not the victim will tell anybody else about it—at work and in social situations he usually won't—he'll tell the doctor. And what Mr. Reis told me served largely to deepen the mystery of why he had headaches.

He was getting headaches, as he'd indicated by his earlier gesture, across the front of his head. They seemed deepest in his forehead just above his right eye. It was a pulsing, throbbing pain that tended to become steady if the headache continued long enough.

We continued to discuss Gunther Reis's headaches. I listened, for I believe that one of the most important aids in attacking the headache is a good and extremely detailed case history of the patient. You may catch anything from the last time he'd had a spinal tap, which sometimes causes headaches, to whether he had hay fever headaches as a child.

You may also learn what has already been done in this case personally and professionally for that matter. I'm against plunging hastily into expensive

6

in-hospital examinations of headache patients if they've had this kind of examination time and again. To be sure, you must check out the patient's organic condition. If he or she hasn't had a checkup recently or is clearly suffering from an organic problem, you must check the patient out thoroughly. But if the patient has had one or two full checkups recently, you stand a chance of doing less for his or her headache than you do to the victim's general outlook. "By the time it's done, the patient may be more disgusted with his physician than with his headache," said the late Donald J. Dalessio, who was a highly respected retired headache expert at the Scripps Clinic and Research Foundation in La Jolla, California. In addition, certain parts of the examination, such as computerized axial tomography (CT) scans and MRI may actually increase the patient's headache, not to mention the effects of the anxiety over the tests. So if a patient has had a full checkup recently, I'll get that patient's records before I would consider hospitalization. Placing a patient in the Diamond Inpatient Unit at Presence St. Joseph Hospital in Chicago with the type of problem exhibited by Gunther Reis enormously increases our success rate, and thus helps the patient by preventing the headache from becoming a chronic problem.

In this case, Gunther Reis had clearly seen another doctor.

"Two of them," he said. "You're the third." That didn't bother me. The patient has the right to seek out another doctor if the first, second, tenth, or eleventh can't help him.

In this case, the first was his longtime physician, who'd put him through a very thorough in-hospital checkup.

"He didn't find anything," said Gunther Reis. Presumably that meant no brain tumor. "But those things can grow," he added, a little stubbornly, as if he feared the thought and yet hated to give it up.

The second doctor had given him an office examination. I would repeat it that day on a more specialized level, just in case he missed something. "It's all in your mind," the doctor had told Gunther Reis. "What he meant was, 'It's all in your imagination,'" said Gunther Reis.

7

I could appreciate his distress. But it is no longer necessary today. In recent years, there's been a surge of interest in headache pain by physicians who believe, as I do, that the pain is real, not imagined, and that if there's a real pain, there's an identifiable reason for it. And if you can identify the reason for it, you may stand a chance of ending the pain, or at least reducing it. And that is the greatest advance in the 3,500 years of recorded medical history of headache pain.

Headache is one of man's oldest complaints. In the most ancient, complete medical book known to exist—the *Ebers Papyrus*, which dates to around 1500 B.C.—there is a mention of a "sickness of half the head," which seems to refer to migraine.

The search for relief from headache may go back even further. Archaeological evidence suggests that trepanning was practiced as far back as the Neolithic era. That is to say, tiny segments of the skull were cut away, perhaps to allow the escape of the "evil demons" which were causing pain in the head. Over the years, every conceivable cure has been tried—wrapping the head in potatoes, wrapping the neck in a hangman's noose, bathing the feet in mustard and farina, sniffing the moss that had grown on a human skull—somebody else's long-unused skull, of course. St. Gregory, who lived in the sixth century, vowed he'd been relieved of a severe headache by pressing his head to the rail around the sepulcher of the tomb of St. Martin.

There are those who look at the proliferation of headaches in our time, particularly among the young, and observe that they are not only symptoms of a sick person but of a sick society, one filled with tension, anxiety, depression, repressed hostilities, frustration—all of which indeed are profoundly involved with one kind of headache pain or another. And yet, we find evidence that the headache was known in the pre-Columbian Peruvian civilization, or the Mesopotamian civilization 3,000 years before Christ, or in the 10th century Arabia, or later in Java or in New Zealand. Clearly, a deeper and more probative understanding of headache pain was needed. And it had to be based on scientific fact, not on centuries of myths. The monumental research of the late Dr. Harold G. Wolff of Cornell Medical College did much to aid our understanding. He found that the brain does not, in itself, hurt; it is in fact insensitive to pain. This remarkable mass of tissue, the body's control center, can be cut, burned, frozen, and probed—all without hurting. So, clearly it is not the brain that hurts in headaches.

What hurts are the nerves and the blood vessels around the brain, the muscles in the head and neck, the meninges (the coverings of the brain)—almost anything but the brain. Different things cause pain in different parts of the brain. One type of headache is concentrated pretty much in the blood vessels when they swell and impinge on the very sensitive nerves; another is concentrated in the muscles when they are pulled terribly taut. Still other types of headaches involve inflammation of the membranes around the brain (meninges).

Another important element in our understanding has been the growing realization that headache pain is a symptom and could be a disease. That symptom, that pain, means there is something wrong. The "something wrong" may be in the organs; it may be anything from arthritis to glaucoma—although I'd estimate that fewer than 2 percent of the headache patients really suffer from an organic problem.

The something wrong may be in the patient's environment. A mechanic working in a poorly ventilated garage in winter might get a headache from the buildup of carbon monoxide. A person working in a munitions plant might get a headache from the nitrate used in the manufacture of high explosives.

In fact, we had a case just like that. It involved a woman in her 50s who began getting the same kind of "migraine attacks" that she used to get when she was a young girl. She couldn't understand this and neither could any of the doctors who treated her. For migraine very seldom lasts beyond menopause and almost never (note I say almost never) starts striking a woman after menopause.

We discovered that she'd never had a migraine in the first place. When she was young, she worked in a munitions plant and got headaches from the nitrate, which did seem very much like migraine attacks. Certain substances cause chemical changes around the brain similar to those caused in migraine. She left work when she married and the headaches disappeared. Some years ago, a psychiatrist might have attributed the disappearance of the headaches to a change in her sex life.

When her children were grown, she went back to work in the same munitions plant, and the headaches returned. That may have vastly confused the psychiatrists but not headache experts. We simply advised her that the headaches would end when she quit her job in the munitions plant. She did quit, and so did the headaches. Later she wrote me that I must "have the powers of a god." Nothing that impressive—just a modern understanding of headache.

The something wrong may also be in the lifestyle of the patient—a wrong direction taken, perhaps, or a wrong pace. The headache becomes an expression of these uncertainties—perhaps a reflection of a long-term depression or subtle sense of stress that finds no other outlets. Because we understand these things, we can do something about the pain in the head and about the thing that causes it.

Another element in the recent understanding is that there are different kinds of headache. For a long while, a chronic, recurring headache was automatically called "migraine." As a matter of fact, about 37 million people in the United States suffer from migraine. Another 100 million suffer from other kinds of headache.

In 1962, a very prestigious committee, recruited and supported by the United States government and directed by individuals in the private sector of medicine, established 15 different broad categories of headaches. In the late 1990s, the International Headache Society published the findings of their Classification Committee in a special issue of the medical journal, *Cephalalgia*, with a more extensive classification of headaches that contained more than 300 pages. This classification has been updated several times since then, and the most recent edition, *The International Classification of Headache Disorders*,

3rd edition (Beta version) was published in 2013. This latest version describes 14 different categories of headache. Basically, this classification is used essentially only for research. Such classifications are vital to the treatment of headache. Obviously, you wouldn't treat the swelling of blood vessels in the head with exactly the same medicine that you'd use to ease the tightening of muscles in the neck and head. But it is very difficult to remember and pinpoint or use 14 different kinds of headache classifications. Accordingly, several of my colleagues and I have tried to simplify the classifications further, if only because identification is so vital in the treatment of headache.

One of the most important decisions in diagnosing a headache patient is determining whether the patient is suffering from a *primary headache* or a *secondary headache*. Primary headaches include migraine, tension-type headache, and cluster headache. Secondary headache can be attributed to another cause, such as a brain tumor or a bleed in the brain. While secondary headaches are, as a group, relatively rare, due to their inherent risks, the physician must first rule these out with a thorough physical examination and, when warranted, imaging.

Further research into headache pain is hindered by obvious difficulties: we cannot open a human head and look inside when a person has pain. Indeed, we cannot easily do it with animals, as we can in research on other ailments, because we cannot readily tell when an animal has a headache pain. But we have been able to work out some procedures for use with headache-racked humans. For example, we can take blood samples when such patients have a headache and when they don't, and this has helped enormously in headache research by enabling us to identify changes in levels of certain chemicals in the blood which take place during a headache.

Yet we are still short of our ultimate goal: we cannot always tell what causes or what cures headache. To be sure, we can "cure" a certain number of headaches. Given the proper circumstances, the easily treated cause behind the symptom, we can completely erase headache pain. But that doesn't happen very often. We don't talk much of cures, and never of miracle cures. We do talk about reducing pain and managing headaches, and even that may take considerable time.

In short, we don't want to inspire over-optimism in our patients. Most of them have had headache pain for a long, long time and most of them understand that they will not end it completely and forever overnight. If they've been made helpless by pain, as many of them have, we can help them to function again as viable, lively, and fulfilled persons, but we cannot promise to end their pain forever.

There is little that is automatic in the treatment of headache pain. Probably there is no other health problem that has been so completely surrounded by as much confusion, worry, and mistreatment as the headache. This has, understandably, jaundiced some patients, and so we, as "experts" in headache, must deal with the patient as well as the pain. Our first effort is, as I've said earlier, to deal with the pain of the headache. Our next effort is to deal with its cause. The search for these solutions often seems like a detective mystery with the doctor sifting through clues, following up leads, poring over evidence. We actually have two mysteries on our hands with each patient: one to see what kind of headache pain it is, the other to find the cause; both are baffling, frustrating, exhilarating. That's why we've presented the case histories in this book in terms of their mystery and their clues, and that's why we started the discussion with the mystery of Gunther Reis.

As my conversation with Gunther Reis continued, I could see how he'd won his success. He was not very much the arbiter of elegance, yet he was so knowing in his responses and so judicious that I could understand how even the graybeards of the advertising game might come to pay him a great deal of respect. Our conversation was not one-way. He was trying to get the matter of the brain tumor resolved immediately.

Doctors do not like to be rushed by patients. Yet I was tempted to respond to Gunther Reis's urgency. He needed a certain amount of assurance.

From this point of view, the tumor—if, indeed, there was one—had been growing for three months and the sooner we got at it the better.

"I can clear the next two days for hospital tests," he said.

"I'm not sure that's necessary," I said. I much preferred to get the results of his recent tests and study them before I put him through yet another battery of hospital tests.

"But why don't I run a series of preliminary tests right now?" I said.

These uncomplicated tests can be performed in the office. They cannot with certainty disclose the presence of a tumor, unless it is very obvious, but they can give very strong evidence that there is none. And they can help to eliminate some of the possibilities of certain organic disturbances.

The tests involved a basic examination of the eyes, the ears, and the nose. They also involved a neurological examination—a series of very simple tests. Some doctors run a scanty neurological test; I prefer a more complete one. It is astonishing what a doctor can learn from watching a patient balance himself, or walk a straight line, or touch fingertip to nose, or a dozen other simple tests. It is revealing to know what can be learned simply by tapping a patient on the knee with a rubber hammer or tickling the soles of his feet and watching which way the toes curl. (One way, the wrong way, can signal some serious problems of the central nervous system or of a particular side of the brain.)

After the tests were conducted, I told him I'd study them and let him know the results at our next appointment. If I'd encountered something serious and significant, I'd have had him in the hospital that night. As it was, I suggested he come back in two weeks.

"Isn't that a bit long?" He had a way of challenging a person with a concentrated stare when he asked a question.

"Come back in a week if you prefer," I said. He couldn't: he'd be on a business trip in a week. So we compromised on 10 days.

"In the meantime, take this medicine," I said. I wrote out a prescription for naproxen sodium. (See Appendix II, Drugs Used in Acute Migraine Attacks.) When he walked out the door, my mind was already filtering through the various clues and alternatives.

Did he have a tension-type headache—one that originated in the psyche and caused a tightening of the muscles in the head and neck? Certainly he was in a profession that could inspire anxiety and when things go wrong, as they often do, could inspire a long-term depression. But Gunther Reis didn't seem to have this kind of depression. He did not suffer from the "hatband" pain—the kind that seems to totally encircle the head—or the duration of pain characteristic of a tension-type headache. His pain came irregularly and lasted for only a portion of the day, while those suffering from tension-type headaches tend to get them virtually every day or at least many days a week, and their headaches never seem to go away.

He did not suffer the kind of sleep disturbances common to tension-type headaches. Patients with headaches due to depression usually wake up very early in the morning and then can't go back to sleep. But Gunther Reis said that he'd been sleeping pretty much as always, and there was nothing in his job situation that indicated an increased anxiety or depression.

To me, that indicated there was little chance he was suffering from a tension-type headache. I did not eliminate it completely—headaches are a very tricky and sometimes you get two or three different types in the same patient—but I was very much inclined to look elsewhere for the cause of his trouble.

Did he have, for instance, an inflammatory headache or one caused by organic problems?

The early tests, in my office, suggested this was not the case. But we'd know more about that after I looked over the reports from his previous doctor and, if he insisted, after we put him through further tests as an inpatient.

Did he have a headache that, after a series of neurological changes, results in the swelling of blood vessels around the brain? That seemed the most

14

likely cause to me. The pain was located in the same place and acted in the ways vascular headaches tend to act. Yet it didn't seem quite like a migraine headache—the most common form of vascular headache. For one thing, migraine rarely begins to attack men of his age; it tends to be much more a headache of the younger years. Also, the headache was not as regular as migraine, and he didn't get the warning signs that patients with migraine with aura (formerly known as classic migraine) get—the aura some 20 or 30 minutes before the pain, for example. But that is not necessarily conclusive; many people get a kind of migraine, called migraine without aura (formerly known as common migraine)—in which these warning signs are absent or imperceptible. In addition, he didn't seem to have the usual "migraine personality." That personality is merely a clue, for a few people with migraine do not exhibit all the most familiar traits of the migraine personality, and many people without migraine do have those characteristics. My strong feeling at the time was to discount migraine but not to eliminate it.

Another kind of headache that, unlike migraine, does strike men more often than women is called a cluster headache, because it occurs in clusters. A victim will get three or four or more headaches every day for several weeks or several months; then the headaches will go away completely for three or four months, only to come back in clusters. They seem, in fact, to be seasonal, and some physicians have mistaken them for anxiety headaches, simply because, coming in the spring, they strike businessmen at income tax or annual report time. Actually, there is no connection between the two; these aren't anxiety headaches. They are a very singular kind of headache.

Again, the matchup was not encouraging. Gunther Reis did not have the characteristic look of the "cluster" victim: the very square-jawed look with the furrowed forehead, the roughened skin on the cheeks, or the overall thick facial skin. He did not have the tears that usually flow from one eye of the cluster victim, or the runny nose. Moreover, his headaches did not seem to come in clusters; he got them irregularly; they did not come at the same time of the day, as clusters seem to do; he sometimes got them early in the morning but more often later in the day. Clusters usually last 60 to 90 minutes, sometimes a little longer, while his seemed to continue for the better part of a day. And there was another more subtle point which those of us who specialize in headache pain have come to observe: cluster victims tend to pace, in an effort to mute their pain, while migraine victims tend to go to bed, in an effort to sleep away their pain. Gunther Reis had said that he went home and went to bed when he had a headache.

So, although cluster seemed the best bet in terms of age and onset, there were just enough factors in the matchup to make me inclined to eliminate it, too. Thus, I suspected three or four kinds of headaches that Gunther Reis didn't have. But I still didn't know the kind of headache he did have.

In a sense, all of medicine is like this. But perhaps the headache field is more like a continuing mystery than any other field, if only because it starts with pain, and pain is very subjective. You can learn about it only from the person suffering it. But there are no hard-and-fast standards as to what pain is. You can't measure it the way you can measure a fever—with a precise number of degrees. Some people, for example, have more resistance to pain than others. Some people have two different kinds of pain, really two different kinds of headaches, but they don't know it. A pain that strikes in the darkest hours of night may seem far more dismaying and have a much more dreadful impact than one that strikes in the daytime. And a pain that can be explained by the victim to himself, such as a hangover headache, is a lot less frightening, if no more comforting, than a pain that is totally inexplicable.

None of this was any consolation to Gunther Reis when he returned for his second visit. He had had another severe attack of headache pain while on a recent business trip to San Francisco.

"Didn't the medicine I prescribed do any good?" (It's important for a doctor to know what won't work as well as what will work.)

He looked embarrassed. "I forgot to pack it," he said.

16

"Did you take aspirin?"

He nodded. "And the sumatriptan. I still had a bottle in a shaving kit." He paused. "But it didn't seem to do much."

All right. Nothing happens perfectly. People forget, even when they have pain. They also hope that they won't need anything for their pain.

If he didn't have anything enlightening to report to me, I didn't have anything to report to him. I'd received and studied the reports of his earlier tests, and there was no indication of any organic disturbance, much less a brain tumor.

He thought it over for a moment. "Let's do it again," he said. "It's been a couple of months since this"—he indicated the report—"and something might show up now that didn't then. Unless you know positively it's because of something else."

Well, I didn't know that positively. In fact, the possibility of organic problems was the only one that I had not personally eliminated, and I had to consider the patient. Although most persons become more upset by the long and uncomfortable examinations involved in a full checkup, there was every reason to believe this man might be relieved.

So he took a few days off from work and checked into the Diamond Headache Unit at Presence St. Joseph Hospital. We administered all the standard diagnostic tests once again. We gave him a complete physical checkup and a very complete neurological examination. We gave him MRI of the brain and MRA of the head. We carried out many different blood analyses. We completely monitored the functions of his vital organs, including heart, liver, and kidneys. We studied his gastrointestinal tract. We gave him a long metabolic test. And when we were finished, we had nothing. He was perfectly healthy, except that he had severe and unexplained pains in his head.

At that point, many physicians - particularly those who do not specialize in the headache—would have quietly given up. They'd be sure "it's all in his head." But that's not the way of the headache specialist. It's our custom and responsibility to hang in there all the way. If the case wasn't difficult, it wouldn't have come to us in the first place. Truth to tell, the patient is usually more discouraged than the doctor; for he has the pain and no reason for it.

Gunther Reis was disheartened. I'm not sure he'd have been pleased if we had found something wrong with him, but at least that would have given him an answer so that we might have been able to correct the problem through medicine or surgery.

Now the question was, where do we go from here?

"Look," I said, "I'm willing to stay with it if you are."

He gestured helplessly. He didn't have much choice, other than to hunt up another doctor and face the possibility of yet another thorough checkup and another disappointment. This kind of option, when faced with a job-shattering life of pain, is not terribly encouraging.

I prescribed a tricyclic antidepressant—Elavil (amitriptyline), which is probably the most utilized medication by headache specialists in the prevention of chronic migraine.

"But I want you to do something for me. Do you keep an office diary?"

The question surprised him, but yes, he did. Many people in his position keep records of their business activities for everything from their boss to their clients for income tax purpose.

"I want you to go back in the headache calendar or diary to two or three weeks before you had the first headache. (See Appendix V, Headache Calendar.) I want you to copy out everything you did from that time to right now." Three or four months of notes would give him something to do and make him feel as if something was happening in the search for the cause of his headache. But it was more than therapy; I was looking for more clues to this mystery.

"Then I want you to keep a headache calendar from this point on in greater detail. (See Appendix V, Headache Calendar.) What you do, where you go when you do it." I knew the office diary was likely to be sketchy, showing only the highlights of his day and referring mostly to his work record. But if he

18

could keep a more complete history from this point on, including details of his personal life, I'd have a better chance to dig up some clues.

"And I'd like to ask you to make one more sacrifice: go through one more full-fledged headache. Tell me when it starts and when it ends, and take the naproxen sodium. And don't forget to put down everything you do during every day: where you eat, what you eat, how long you sleep, what clothes and what fabrics you wear, whether you take cabs or park your car in an underground garage, everything."

"Including sex?" he asked with a small smile.

Now sex can be important in breaking the mystery of headache pain. I've had patients who felt intense headache pain during and after sexual intercourse because of an aneurysm enlarging in their brain, or because of high blood pressure. I even had a patient in whom sex inspired anxiety headaches. But Gunther Reis did not suffer from these problems; his checkup proved that conclusively, and I'm not much for voyeurism.

"You can skip the sex," I said.

"Okay. I'll have the office history ready for you as soon as possible. I'll mail it in. How long before I come back with the current history?"

"A month," I said. I saw him flinch. A month more of pain is not a pleasant thought. "But if the headaches get overpowering, give me a phone call. Day or night." This is an arrangement I have with all my patients. "We'll see what can be done then."

In 10 days, the copy of the office history arrived, with his particular notation of what days he'd suffered headaches. The material held a clue—and he must have known it. For the notes showed he usually got the headaches when out of town on business or just after returning to town. Interestingly, some of the trips involved what appeared to be further success in his business. And for a moment I thought that significant.

Some people function well—completely free of headache—under great pressure of business, then seem to suffer headache once they know that success has been assured.

But as it turned out, this wasn't the answer to Gunther Reis's headaches. He got them on certain other business trips that had no great importance to him. They were simply taken as a service to a client or to maintain contacts with a client. So there was no repressed anxiety involved in them. Nevertheless, we had something more to talk about, something significant to explore.

Yet when he came to see me, he was not as expectant as I'd thought. "I thought we had something in the out-of-town trips, too," he said. "Particularly when I got them two more times after out-of-town trips this month." He paused. "I'm not sure I could give the trips up; they're important to my business. Now it doesn't matter. Two other times in the last month, I've had headaches when I didn't leave town. So now I'm getting them whether I leave town or not."

"I'll have a look at the diary anyway," I said. In the meantime, I asked about how the medicine worked, and then changed the prescription slightly. And come back and see me next week."

In that week, I cross-referenced the habits reflected in his diary. One thing turned up repeatedly; both times he'd gone out of town, he'd gone to a Chinese restaurant on the night before returning home. More importantly, both times he got headaches at home was the the day after he'd been to a Chinese restaurant.

That sent me to my reference books. I knew what I was looking for, but I wanted to nail down the "whys." Many people are sensitive to certain elements in Chinese foods, sometimes it is the ingredients in soy sauce, more often to monosodium glutamate (MSG), used as a flavor enhancer in won ton soup and many other Chinese dishes. That sensitivity is a change in the chemicals in the blood that might cause blood vessels in the cranium to swell.

20

"You like Chinese food?" I asked when he came for his next appointment.

"Very much," he said. "Though I've just gotten into it."

"Take a look at the way these references come together." I showed him the key—his visits to a Chinese restaurant on the day before the onset of his headaches, whether he was on or off the road.

"Now can you remember if you ate at Chinese restaurants in those previous three months? In the office diary you didn't have any details of where you ate, unless it was an expense account, on those earlier road trips."

"I'm sure I did. I have certain Chinese restaurants I go to whenever I visit New York or San Francisco. I know I went to them on those earlier trips out of town. And there are one or two places in town I like very much."

"How long have you been doing this? All your life?"

"Oh no. Just the last three or four months."

So now the pattern was complete. He'd gotten headaches at about the same time he started eating Chinese food. And we knew that certain elements in Chinese food cause a reaction in people who are sensitive to them that might involve headache pain.

"So this means I have to give up eating Chinese?" he asked.

"Not necessarily," I said. "This is circumstantial evidence. We can establish proof by having you run through extensive sensitivity tests. Or we can try our own little tests."

"Such as?"

"The next time you go to a Chinese restaurant, have the won ton soup but not the soy sauce. If you get a headache, let me know. After that, we'll try the opposite: have the soy sauce but not the won ton soup. That way we'll eliminate one or the other.

He did exactly as I suggested. He got the headache when he had the won ton soup but not the soy sauce. He got no headache the other way around.

21

"So it looks like the monosodium glutamate triggers migraine in you," I said. "Just be careful and start asking questions. You may find that other Chinese foods—the vegetables, I've heard—are sometimes seasoned with MSG, so you may want to skip them. Just ask questions about any synthetic seasoning you get on any foods anywhere. A good deal of it has MSG in it." And then I ticked off some examples for him: Japanese teriyaki, chicken soup, matzo ball soup, even green pea soup.

I took him off Elavil and asked him to come back in another month. I wanted to make sure no side effects developed as well as any headaches. After that month, he reported fit and happy and said he'd been headache-free since our last talk. The strain, the vaguely haunted look, was gone from his face. His eyes were no longer dark and deep. He was a man who no longer had a worry about the function or the worth of life.

In retrospect, I have to say that it was a rewarding case, but not a miraculous cure. It involved what every headache case involves: a long, scrupulous, often baffling hunt for the cause of the headache and a way to end it. It also involved something which few headache cases involve: a sudden and complete end to headache pain. After you read the rest of this book, you'll begin to appreciate just how rare an event that was.

2

THE CONQUERED PAIN

Her life was, on the surface, the envy of her friends. She lived in a well-to-do suburb with neat lawns and colonial-style homes. She had six children, a husband who was much respected in his field, an unquestioning faith in everything from God to politics, and an ambition that was as resourceful as a squirrel at the onset of winter.

But from the age of 22—six weeks after her marriage—an unforeseen and incomprehensible curse had been laid upon her. She suffered migraine headaches.

"I did have headaches before that—severe headaches," said Jo Hepburn. "But I never had migraine." She picked her words with deliberation and precision, like a party to a case in court who must make her case now or never. "They [the previous headaches] would be in the middle of my head instead of on one side. And they would last—um, I would have a good night's sleep and they'd be gone the next day. But with a migraine, I would go at least three days before I'd get rid of it. I'd be in bed at least a day and a half. After the children came—well, it was very difficult to stay in bed."

Earlier I mentioned that at least 37 million people in the United States have migraine headaches. I feel that I should emphasize that "at least." If that's the case, consider the misery that this company shares.

"I never knew when they would come," said Jo Hepburn, "or what brought them on. They would just suddenly be there. I would get one between [menstrual] periods and often with a period. I would have at least two a month and sometimes I'd get one every 10 days."

She was a slender woman, trim and neatly groomed. She had attractive and competent features—quite a good face, triangular, a lot of bone, and not much flesh. She was practical and sensible, and there was a look in her eyes and

23

about her mouth that indicated a flat-out no-nonsense determination that remained even when she relaxed.

"I think the biggest, most awful thing to live with in a migraine," she continued, "is the feeling that you're very inadequate, that you are being defeated by a headache. There's something wrong with you—and you've got to go to bed. It's very depressing. You're depressed all the time because you're sick and you've been defeated."

She had a case of migraine with aura. That put her in a small minority of migraine sufferers—perhaps 10 to 20 percent of the total. The remainder experience migraine without aura, which lacks some or many of the characteristics of migraine with aura. But Jo Hepburn had them all; there was never any doubt about her problem.

Some of the indications are described in the following paragraph. *She was getting a distinct aura about a half-hour before the pain. "I would see dots," she said. "I would see little dots. My eyes would bother me terribly in the light. And I'd get a funny taste in my mouth." All things considered, this was a tolerable aura. In some cases, to speak of the aura is to call up the macabre: all caves and grottoes, the circle and amphitheaters of hell, the rites of barbarians in a dark forest. Some people see stars flashing as brightly as the sun; some see figures and fortifications out of a medieval nightmare; some see a rainbow or halo over a human figure; one or two out of history interpreted their auras as visions that were divinely inspired. A few people, who have hallucinatory migraine, see only the most grotesque and bizarre. Some authorities claim that Lewis Carroll, who apparently suffered from hallucinatory migraine, was inspired by his aura to describe Alice in her various incarnations in Alice in Wonderland.*

Aura may be manifested in various ways. Some patients may suffer either a partial or near-total loss of vision. Some feel that the illumination in the room is at fault; you'll sometimes see migraine victims take off their spectacles and polish them in the minutes before a headache comes on. In some patients, other senses are affected. I once had a patient whose sense of smell was profoundly affected—for the worse. Before she got a migraine pain, she smelled a terrible and most repulsive odor in her own body. The odor wasn't real—it was due to a distortion of her sense of smell caused by migraine—but of course she didn't know that. She genuinely thought her body smelled bad. And since she didn't know when the migraine and the odor might strike, she withdrew more and more from public and personal contact for fear of embarrassing her friends and herself. She became, in fact, a recluse because of the distortion of the olfactory sense brought on by the migraine. It was not until she came to us for the pain and we explained that the smell was not real—it was as imagined as a visual hallucination—that she began to emerge from her self-imposed isolation.

Jo Hepburn had a family history of migraine. Her aunt and her cousin had them, and so did her sister. She believed that two of her children—one 14 and one 20—also had them.

A family history of migraine is believed to be highly significant in reaching a diagnosis. In 1954, Dr. Harold Wolff[1] and two of his colleagues published a study of 199 individuals with chronic headache and they found three things about the connection of migraine in families: (1) 69.2 percent of those persons in the study whose parents both had migraine also had migraine; (2) 44.2 percent of those who had one parent with migraine had it; (3) 28.6 percent of those whose parents didn't have migraine but who had some other relative with migraine, such as an aunt or a cousin, had it.

Another researcher who studied husband-and-wife combinations with migraine found 91 percent of the parents of these couples had experienced

---

[1] Dr. Harold Wolff was a distinguished professor and chairman of the Department of Neurology and Internal Medicine at Cornell University in the 1950s and '60s. He was so dynamic that he refused to take the specialty exams in neurology because he felt no one was capable of testing him. He did experiments in the 1950s that no ethical committee or experimental committee would have permitted. He did craniotomies on patients during migraine attacks to observe what was happening visually.

migraine attacks, and 83 percent of the children of these couples also had migraine attacks. Jo Hepburn also had what I've already described as a migraine personality. This was first defined in 1937 by Dr. Wolff. Generally, he described migraine sufferers' personalities as being perfectionist, orderly, ambitious, cautious, and emotionally constipated; that is, they repress emotions, such as anger or hostility or a sense of explosions. By and large, they are also very bright and alert (Thomas Jefferson, John Calvin, St. Paul, and Sigmund Freud were migraine sufferers); they talk very quickly and to the point, and they tend to overload or to expect too much of themselves. Now this is not to say that every one of the millions of people who have migraine is exactly like this. Nor is it to say the opposite—that everybody who is like this has migraine. We all know exceptions. I know one energetic, bright, driven woman, as chirpy as a bird, who shows no signs of migraine. And I have friends who say that I am driven, ambitious, overloaded in my work, talk very fast, and that I am somewhat picky and precise. I file away every relevant piece of paper that I come across, and yet I don't have migraine. My point is that you look for a migraine personality in people who have a pain in their heads and you won't always be misled. But the personality is only the general clue, not a final index of what the pain is all about.

In Jo Hepburn, the general migraine personality was pronounced, though not in every final detail. "When it comes to doing housework, no, I'm not a perfectionist," she said. "Certainly, there are things that will just drive me crazy, like clutter and dirty windows, when it comes to doing housework. But there are some things I can live with for years. Dust on something—on top of a picture frame—and I'll never see it. But there are things that drive me out of my mind—like dirty dishes in the sink, I can't stand them."

Similarly, she denied that she was overloaded with activities—other than bearing five children in her first six years of marriage. When she lived in Buffalo, she was in a church-action group and she served on the bishop's committee for the mothers of preschool children. When the family moved to

26

Omaha, she was not only active in church groups but in conservative politics and in writers' groups. When the family moved to Chicago, she took on all this and a little bit more. She began writing children's books.

She was doing all this with all the children and with headaches that were sending her to bed for three to nine days a month. Yet her compulsive drive was so great that she would never admit that she might be overloaded.

"No, because I would never admit that I couldn't do whatever I wanted to do," she said. "That was part of my makeup. Perhaps it was something I should have tried to overcome. But I always felt that I could do whatever I wanted to do and there was no amount of work, nothing that could be put in my path that I couldn't overcome. This is probably why those headaches were so frustrating, and why I hated to admit to anyone that I had them. They were a sign of weakness, and I didn't like that in me.

At first, the headaches came any time of the day or night. "But later on, as I got older, they seemed to come on weekends quite often." "Older" meant in her 30s; she was only in her late 30s when I first saw her. "Not always, but quite often they would come on weekends, until it got to be a very depressing thing and I began to expect them on a weekend. I often wondered if the mere expectation didn't cause it."

Dr. Oliver Sacks, an eminent medical writer and friend, recently deceased, has reported on a 35-year-old engineer, a brilliant and insatiably ambitious man, who worked day and night, including all evenings and all weekends, to make a success of the think tank he'd started. (It offered computing and mathematical research work to private industry.) Suddenly, he began waking up every Sunday morning with an increasingly severe migraine headache. (The suddenness was unusual, but migraine will attack a man in his 30s.) At first, he forced himself to work through Sunday despite the migraine, but eventually he fell so seriously ill with nausea and vomiting that he had to take the day off and spend it in bed.

Here was a man, suggests Dr. Sacks, who, if it were humanly possible, would have worked 24 hours a day, 7 days a week, 168 hours a week. But it was not humanly possible, and so he developed migraine-on-Sunday, one which sent him to bed, possibly as a warning he was overloading himself. The regular migraine-on-Sunday became a sort of psychological Sabbath that forced him to take the needed rest usually dictated by religious custom or good sense. It was the only way his body and his nervous system could get any rest. In my experience, sleep will help a migraine attack, so many migraineurs will go to bed at the first sign of an attack.

Whether Jo Hepburn got migraine on weekends or at other times, she did not let her friends and guests know. She did the best she could while never mentioning her affliction.

"I was ashamed," she said, "Any migraine victim will tell you they're ashamed of it . . . I felt like a complete neurotic. I felt that there was something wrong with me mentally for me to be completely bedridden by nothing more than a headache."

Though her friends did not often know she suffered from migraine, her family did. And they had to adjust to the problem.

"They were always very good when they knew I had a headache," she said. "I'd wait a long time before I'd tell them. Because I was embarrassed. I was ashamed. So I'd wait and wait, hoping I'd get through the day and they could get to bed before I'd admit that I had a headache."

"They would help. As they got older, they would do what they could to help." The oldest of the children was 21 when I first saw Jo Hepburn. Then they came in at 20, 18, 17, and 15. And finally the sixth child, who would be 10 that summer.

"And Joe [her husband] was always good. When he came home from work, he would take over. So I can't say the family ever did or said anything, but in a very minor way: 'Oh, you've got a headache again.'"

28

So it was her problem and the family accepted it as such. But she felt it in many dimensions. "The only thing was that it was enough to make me feel guilty. There was a lot of guilt feeling," she said. "But I can never blame my family for looking upon these headaches as something that . . . they never insinuated that there was something wrong with me, other than that there was a headache. It was all my own feeling.

"I tried various ways to get rid of it. But it never went away. I'd try to relax, try to talk myself out of it, tell myself that I really wasn't getting a headache, that was all in my head.

"But it didn't work. It was all in my head, but it didn't work. I got to the point of depression and despair; it was an awful feeling."

When headaches like Jo Hepburn's continue for 15 years or more, they have considerable impact on the attitudes of their victims. Pain literally dominates their lives. They can get nobody else to understand quite how bad it is, while they surrender time and time again to the tyranny of pain.

"I wasn't living," said Jo Hepburn. "I was existing—from day to day, week to week—wondering if this was the day, this was the weekend that was going to be it. I could plan nothing. I could count on nothing."

Of course she went to the doctor. Time and again. In one city after another.

"When we lived in Buffalo, the doctor there would give me various painkillers. They never worked. Then we moved to Omaha and I just continued using—well, I didn't really get any help from that doctor there. And then we moved to Chicago, my doctor was not at all concerned. That is a problem I found with doctors; they didn't understand headaches. A headache, they said, was something that everybody got once in a while and you had to learn to cope with it. And if you couldn't, well that was too bad. They had too many other and more important things to worry about than headaches. They just didn't really care."

Did all this tend to leave her feeling defeated?

29

"Oh yes, yes. Not only defeated but that there was really no answer, and that I never could find an answer. Because no doctor really cared that much. They were doing—well, there was no research on migraine that I knew of at the time and, as I say, it just wasn't that important to most doctors. They had people with heart attacks and high blood pressure and kidney disease and everything else to worry about—much more serious supposedly. But I feel that migraine can be extremely serious. At least when it takes so much of your life."

It happened that at the time Jo Hepburn came in, I'd received a grant to conduct research into migraine. I needed the help of a good many migraine patients in order to carry out the research, and I had no place to get them. Research facilities don't have migraine victims stored up on lists and hospitals, as they have cancer or heart victims.

So within the limits demanded by my profession, I put a personal classified ad in a Chicago newspaper asking for people who had what they thought were migraine headaches to call my office. Advertising for research patients wasn't typically done back then, but I hoped to find enough genuine sufferers to carry out the migraine study. That probably wouldn't work today as people depend on the Internet and Facebook more. Today, researchers spend enormous amounts of money on TV, radio, and large ads in publications. Jo Hepburn was one of the people who saw my ad.

Her problem, migraine, was known for thousands of years before it was labeled. And, if the evidence from the Neolithic age is any indication, it has been known for hundreds of thousands of years. Galen, the Greek physician of the second century after Christ, wrote some 83 treatises that still exist, and in one of them he told of a one-sided pain in the head which he called hemicrania—hemi, "one-half," crania meaning "the head." You could see how the "mi" and the "graine" developed out of that term.

The pain, as is apparent from the phrase, is one-sided most of the time. In migraine with aura, it hits on the side opposite the side on which the aura is seen, often just behind the eyebrow. (In migraine without aura, the pain may turn up on either side of the head; indeed, sometimes it occurs first on one side, later on the other side.) The pain is dull—in contrast to the very sharp pain of a cluster headache—and throbbing. If the headache lasts long enough, the pain becomes constant.

We've noted three and four famous individuals who suffered from migraine. Actually, there are many, many more: Frederic Chopin, Charles Darwin, Leo Tolstoy, Alfred Nobel, Karl Marx, Edgar Allen Poe, Peter Illich Tchaikovsky, and Virginia Woolf. It is said that Queen Mary Tudor—"Bloody Mary"—went to her coronation with a migraine. And that General Ulysses S. Grant, a chronic headache victim, suffered an agonizing migraine for two days in the wilderness before Appomattox, and then felt the headache disappear swiftly when he received a note from Robert E. Lee asking for a meeting at Appomattox Court House. (As we shall see, a crisis is one way of attacking migraine pain.)

The only way we can explain migraine in so many famous and accomplished people is by referring back to some of the elements in the migraine personality: these people are very bright and alert. They are the "doers." They are utterly determined that they are going to achieve a particular goal at a particular time and nothing, not even a severe and recurring headache, is going to stop them.

Note that there was a good many men on that list of celebrated migraine sufferers. This is unusual. Not because men aren't achievers, but because, statistically, men are a small minority of the migraine sufferers.

Estimates vary but it is believed 60 to 80 percent of all migraine sufferers are women. This may be because the balance of female hormones—as in the menstrual cycle, in pregnancy, and in menopause—is implicated in the cycle of migraine. Or it may be because men simply won't report migraine pain as readily as women will, that they think it is a sign of weakness or something that they can "break through" with their masculine determination. Eventually, perhaps, they will realize that there's nothing they alone can do to conquer the

31

pain. They will have to admit they have it and go to a doctor to try to get something done about it. If that happens, we might find the statistics that migraine is a pain that knows no gender.

In migraine, a series of neurological changes occur that eventually lead to the blood vessels in the cranium to swell. The pain is often throbbing due to the natural pulsations that we all have in our cerebrospinal fluid (CSF), which is the protective liquid that surrounds our brain and spinal cord. When a person is experiencing a migraine attack, the swollen blood vessels, together with central sensitization - when higher order neurons, or nerve cells, become active and normal stimuli can become painful, lead these pulsations to cause pain.

Logic suggests that something must be happening besides the swelling of the blood vessels of the head. If you sit in a very hot bath, the blood vessels in your head will swell, but you won't suffer a pain like migraine. If you exercise long and hard, your blood vessels will swell without causing pain.

That's what makes some of us feel that the blood vessels not only swell but become inflamed in some way. We suspect it is a sterile inflammation; the blood vessels become inflamed but not infected. (When you have a cut or a pimple and the skin around the sore becomes very red, inflamed, it is usually infected, too.) We believe the inflammation as well as the pressure on distended walls of the blood vessels, together with central sensitization, cause the pain.

We know what causes the blood vessels to begin swelling and become inflamed. Changes take place in the amines (histamine and serotonin prominent among them), neuropeptides (including calcitonin gene related peptide, or CGRP, which has become the focus in the development of the newest medications to treat migraine), the catecholamines, the peptide kinins, the prostaglandins, and an acidic lipid called SRSA.

One of the reasons I mention them is to help you understand what's going on during a migraine. Take one example: we know that serotonin, which is given off by the platelets (blood cells) is deeply implicated in migraine. One kind of change in serotonin causes the blood vessels around the brain to constrict, letting less blood through. That's what happens at the start of a migraine episode when you begin seeing an aura; there is less blood, and thus less oxygen is getting through to the brain and many strange things begin happening to the senses (including a partial or total shutoff of vision).

But then, very curiously, another change involving serotonin takes place, and the blood vessels no longer constrict. Instead, they begin dilating, or swelling, and that's when the aura stops and the pain begins.

Now comes the baffling point: We know what changes are taking place, but we don't know why they are taking place. This is an area where a good deal of research is now underway that has led to the development of an exciting group of medications that target CGRP, the neuropeptide mentioned earlier. This neuropeptide plays an integral role in the dilation of blood vessels, and through blocking the action of CGRP, these medications can inhibit the blood vessels from dilating, thus effectively preventing a migraine attack from occurring.

Research of brain chemistry has indicated that with depression chemicals called neurotransmitters—serotonin, norepinephrine, and others—become depleted. These chemicals are necessary for the nervous system to communicate the nerve impulses properly from one cell to the next. When these chemicals are not present, the nervous system cannot perform its functions properly. Furthermore, depending on which areas of the brain are affected, this can cause disturbances of sleep, appetite, and so forth. Pain can result from this as well, and it may be the reason patients with depression have chronic headache. Interestingly, in migraine headache, this depletion of neurotransmitters also appears to occur with each migraine headache attack. (Some recent work from Denmark has challenged our previous concepts about migraine, the premise being that migraine is primarily a neurogenic disease.) A theory of spreading depression across the brain cortex has become very prevalent and believed by many to be the primary cause of migraine associated with the chemical changes in the blood.

Some of the chemical changes seem to be related to the menstrual cycle. Indeed, a great many migraine attacks are associated with the menstrual cycle. Moreover, some 80 percent of women who have migraine stop having migraine headaches from the end of the second month of pregnancy until delivery. About 75 percent, perhaps more, of all migraine headaches disappear after menopause.

The one thing that is common to all these events is a dramatic change in the hormonal balance of the female body. It may be that a lowering of levels of the female hormones, estrogen and progesterone, also lowers the incidence of migraine and raising them increases the chance of migraine.

This theory is supplemented by the effects of the birth control pill on certain women: they get migraine more often and more intensely than ever before. The Pill changes the hormone balance, causing levels of estrogen to rise.

Now a very logical next question is this: How does a hormonal change in the body cause changes in the substances around the brain that in turn cause the blood vessels first to constrict and then to dilate?

We don't altogether know the answer to that. But even if we did, we'd have several points still open to question. For this does not altogether explain why men, small children, or even infants, get migraine. It's my belief that the monthly alterations in the women's hormones in women act as a trigger for them to get more attacks.

Or consider other chemical events in the body. We know, for example, that drinking red wine and eating aged cheese, nuts, freshly baked bread, lima beans, navy beans, yogurt, vinegar (except white vinegar), pork, citrus fruit, onions, herring, and certain other foods—anything fermented, pickled, or marinated—tends to touch off a migraine headache. We also know that the one substance all these foods have in common is a chemical called tyramine. We know finally that tyramine tends to set into motion certain hormonal and circulatory changes in the body. But we still don't know exactly why it might cause those substances in or around the brain to act as they do in migraine. It's

34

been my clinical impression that only 30-40 percent of migraineurs are helped by diet. (See Appendix VI, The Diamond Headache Clinic's Dietary Plan for Headache Patients.)

And even if we did know, there is no one among us who'd dare say, "Just don't eat cheese and port and freshly baked bread or drink red wine every night and your headaches will go away forever." For some migraine, or perhaps most of it, would go on and on. (But one thing I will say: If a migraine sufferer avoids these foods and drink, he'll stand a good chance of reducing the frequency and intensity of the pain.)

There are other routes to consider. We know that certain kinds of stress, such as great fear or suddenly inspired excitement, cause an increase in adrenaline in the body. Other kinds of stress may cause other chemical changes that bring about migraine attacks. Such stress may be slower burning than the adrenaline episodes, for example, the stress of adjusting to a new job, or of living in a new city, or even fatigue, hunger, eyestrain, or the pressure of preparing for a big party. If we knew precisely whether and what kind of stress caused certain changes in the substances around the brain, we might have a clue as to how to control migraine—either by controlling the chemical change or by controlling the stress.

Or consider other forms of emotional reaction: they, too, may cause certain actions and reactions, even chemical ones, in the body that lead to migraine. Repressed emotions are often associated with migraine. In his book *Migraine...Understanding a Common Disorder* (University of California Press, 1985), Dr. Oliver Sacks cites the case of a 44-year-old man who had been employed for many years by an uncle whom he loathed. The uncle did everything possible to humiliate the man, often making sarcastic remarks publicly about his work, but the pay was far better than he would receive in a comparable job elsewhere. Thus he was reluctant to leave for what would certainly be lower pay. His reaction went in another direction. Two or three times a week he would get severe migraine attacks, but only during his working year. When he was on vacation, he'd be completely free of headache pain.

Now this is only circumstantial evidence, although it is powerful and persuasive. It's possible that there were other factors in this man's life which caused or contributed to his migraine. But the indication is strong that he was suffering a deep rage over his humiliating circumstances—over being in bondage to a cruel uncle—and that instead of yelling and screaming at his uncle, he repressed his rage and converted it into migraine headaches instead.

We can know all that and still not know quite how that repressed rage is expressed chemically within the body in a way that causes those substances near the brain to touch off migraine.

Those of us in headache research have seen the family factor over and over again throughout our careers, and now we have genetic evidence to support these observations. Genetic mutations have been identified that are responsible for a severe type of migraine known as familial hemiplegic migraine. Families with these genetic mutations have been found to have up to a 98 percent penetrance (meaning nearly all offspring from individuals with this mutation are afflicted with this condition. It is probable that in the coming years additional genetic evidence will be uncovered to support the assumption that most migraine does indeed carry with it a genetic component.

One strong school of thought asserts that migraine might well be the result of a hereditary chemical imbalance that produces the needed biochemical changes in the body and in the substances around the brain when a susceptible individual is placed in a "triggering" situation; for example, as a result of stress.

In addition to the neuropeptide CGRP discussed earlier, another chemical many researchers tend to identify as a migraine trigger is serotonin, and they focus on the way in which it is metabolized by the body; that is, how the body handles the substance. In fact, Dr. Dalsgaard T. Nielsen of Denmark, one of the most notable figures in headache research in the world, took a poll of all the available headache experts throughout the world and found that most believed migraine to be an inherited disorder that somehow affected the serotonin metabolism of the body.

There is still another possibility: that migraine is a genetic disorder; that it is transmitted through a gene. The theory here is that a gene, passed down through family lines, cause migraine or at least an inclination to migraine in certain people when those people encounter a triggering situation—stress, hormonal changes, such as those caused by the Pill or menstruation, or perhaps certain foods. Moreover, it is within the nature of the genetic code to flash the migraine signal at a certain time. Some people may get the migraine signal in infancy, others in puberty; still others might not get it until their early thirties.

The genetic theory helps to explain a great deal about migraine: why men and women get it, why infants as well as adults get it, why so many different and totally unrelated factors seem to stimulate it, why there is a family factor beyond parent and child.

Even if the theory eventually turns out to be fact, there is one very large problem: it's difficult to cure a genetic disorder. You just can't pull out the genes causing migraine at will. You must first identify the particular gene and see how it works. Even then, you may not be able to do anything in this generation but can hope only to prevent its being passed on to the next generation. So the overall cure for migraine will not suddenly appear if and when we find out that migraine is genetic disorder. A migraine-specific chromosome has been identified, however it has not led to any breakthroughs in treatment.

From all this, you can see that there are no final answers for the cure of migraine. Indeed, we know a lot of things that are involved in migraine, but we still don't know its total and singular cause, or indeed if there is one. But fortunately, we don't need to know the single precise end cause of migraine in order to begin attacking the pain. There are certain drugs that will simply kill pain. There are other drugs that will prevent the blood vessels from swelling, or prevent the change in a substance such as serotonin from taking place, and thus prevent the migraine from taking place. And beyond all this, there are ways that a migraine sufferer can manage his or her life to reduce the pain and the frequency of migraine.

None of these methods will necessarily lead to a final and permanent cure in any one patient. But then you've got to believe that a person who has suffered from severe headaches for 10 or 20 years doesn't really expect a doctor to end them overnight. He or she merely expects the doctor to care about ending them and to carry on a course of treatment that not only promises relief but shows some signs of achieving it. In 2017, *The New Yorker* magazine featured Dr. Elizabeth Loder, an extremely talented headache specialist at Harvard, in an article entitled "The Heroism of Incremental Care." Her treatment of a chronic migraine patient over the course of four years helped him to gradually improve his function. Four years after starting to work with Dr. Loder, the patient was quoted, "I'm a changed person. Dr. Loder saved my life." Migraines had "ruled his life for more than four decades," the author observed.[2] This is the style of headache treatment that I pioneered when I first began treating headache patients.

"I was two-and-a-half years under a doctor's care before I really got some help," said Jo Hepburn. "I mean help that stopped the headache."

That's a long time to keep going to a doctor without getting relief from headache pain. One of the reasons she continued with me, she said candidly, was because she was so desperate, and because she felt that I'd keep after the pain, that I wouldn't give up on her because she had what people called "a mere headache."

It's nothing extraordinary on my part: it's my responsibility. Beyond that, I really believe that it's possible to reduce pain significantly, to the point where the victim can feel she's functioning again in life, as long as the patient is willing to give up the pain. In certain somber circumstances, as you'll see a little later, there are some patients who say they'd like to get rid of the pain but who

[2] A. Gawande, "The Heroism of Incremental Care," *The New Yorker*, January 23, 2017

don't really want to give up certain things built into their lifestyle that involve the pain—such as the tyranny over other members of the family that pain gives them.

With Jo Hepburn, I started with some drugs of an experimental nature. She came to me, after all, in response to a plea for help in a research program. These experimental drugs must be administered only under rigid guidelines set up by the U.S. Food and Drug Administration (FDA). The patient must know that she is receiving an experimental drug, and she must know precisely what its purpose is and how, if at all, it can help her.

Fortunately, Jo Hepburn was so intelligent and verbal that she was an ideal subject. She could follow directions in great detail, and she could report back precisely what the effects and the side effects of the drug were. In this case, there was no effect at all. The drug in question did absolutely nothing to help her. So we went to some of the other drugs available, trying different combinations, in different dosages, and through different methods of administration.

Medications will often undergo several years of use for other medical conditions before being used in migraine patients. In the case of ergot, the drug went through a good many incarnations before it was made fit for use by migraine patients as ergotamine tartrate. Today the most common use of ergot at the Diamond Headache Clinic is in the inpatient unit in the form of dihydroergotamine. Originally, ergot was a fungus growing on rye and, if consumed in its original form, it was a poison. A chemical alloy had to be found for it so that humans could take it without danger. Now it is possible to combine ergot with caffeine. (Caffeine also constricts the blood vessels, and the combination of the caffeine with the ergot, in a compound called Cafergot, seems to have more of an effect than if either one or the other was taken on its own.) It is also possible to combine ergot with certain belladonna alkaloids to help counter intestinal upheaval, or with certain sedatives or barbiturates to help the patient sleep off an attack.

In its various forms, ergot can be taken orally, through a suppository (rectally), intranasal, or it can be injected either intramuscular or intravenous.

Just which way the doctor chooses depends on the circumstances. Injection gets the drug working against the migraine pain faster than any other way, but the patient is not likely to be able to get to the doctor's office to get an injection. Using tablets is the most convenient way, though not the fastest. But if the patient suffers from nausea and vomits as the headache comes on, he may not be able to keep the tablet down. Suppositories are a swift way of getting the medicine into the system, but that is not always the most convenient way; if a person is on a subway train when migraine comes on, he'll definitely prefer a tablet.

Even while you're figuring out which is the best way to administer the medicine, you've got to be calculating the dosage. I tend to be a low-dosage person. I start with the minimum possible dosage to find out if it works, then move up to a slightly higher dosage if it doesn't. Eventually I hope to find a dosage that works without causing any side effects in the patient. (Ergot, for example, should be used cautiously, or not at all, in patients who have cardiac or circulatory problems; it can cause a decrease in the circulation of blood in the hands and legs.)

And then you have to consider both drug and dosage in terms of whether you want to stop the migraine attack as it's coming on or whether you want to prevent it even having a chance of getting started. If it's the former, you want the patient to take the drug as the attack starts and hope that it does the job. If it's the latter, you want the patient to be taking medicine every day or every few hours. My own feeling is to instruct patients to take drugs on a daily basis if they suffer from more than two severe episodes a month. Otherwise I try to work out a discipline that will allow them to try to overcome the headache when it starts.

All this has to be considered in prescribing one drug. When you consider all the possibilities, the right drug in the right combination in the right

40

dosage with the right way of administering it, you can see why it sometimes takes a while to find the right treatment for the right person.

In the 1970s, the scientists at Glaxo in the United Kingdom began investigation on trying to identify the serotonin receptor type responsible for the beneficial effects of serotonin. But the research team led by Patrick Humphrey discovered a receptor type 5-HTIB which mainly affects the cranial blood vessels rather than the peripheral blood vessels. In 1988, the prototype triptan, sumatriptan, was administered by injection and it demonstrated its efficacy and tolerance in treating acute migraine attacks. Subsequent to this, many forms of the drug and methods of administration were discovered by multiple pharmaceutical companies.

The first bit of progress with Jo Hepburn was in attacking her morning migraine. "I would go to bed at night feeling fine," she said, "but I'd wake up the next morning with a terrible headache." We got that under control, but we didn't have the rest of her headache pattern conquered. The mystery was not what was wrong with Jo Hepburn but how to find the right combination that would overcome her problem. "It must have been a year later," she said, "that I got started on Nardil."

Nardil is a trade name for phenelzine sulfate, a monoamine oxidase (MAO) inhibitor. Monoamine oxidase inhibitors (MAOIs) have been used by many doctors to relieve a long-enduring depression in certain patients. But one of my colleagues in Australia, Dr. James W. Lance, found it was also successful in overcoming intractable migraine; that is, a very stubborn migraine which does not yield to other treatment. It reduces, but does not end, the headaches. Usually, it cuts their frequency and their severity in half.

To use the MAOI effectively, the patient must be able to understand instructions and be adherent. She or he must avoid certain foods: cheese, nuts, herring, freshly baked breads, chicken livers, wine, and liquor—(See Appendix VII, The Nardil Diet—When Taking Monoamine Oxidase Inhibitors.) very much the same list of foods that seem to inspire migraine attacks. Now I'd have

41

expected Jo Hepburn to avoid these foods anyway; it simply makes good sense, and I urge this adherence with all my migraine patients. But for those on the MAOI, it is absolutely necessary to avoid these foods, for the drug, in combination with the food, sometimes inspires a very severe, even critical attack of high blood pressure. It might even cause a stroke. During treatment with an MAOI, the patient must not drink any alcohol, including wine. Also, when taking MAOIs, patients must avoid taking any type of decongestant medication and any medicines that have an effect on blood pressure.

I explained to Jo Hepburn, as I do to all my patients, exactly what she was getting in the way of medication—what the medicine was, and how much of it she would be taking. We always tell patients about the medicine. It's my philosophy that people should know what they are getting in the way of medication and why the medication is expected to work. I think people are intelligent enough to know why they are getting a particular drug and what its consequences might be. Beyond this, there's a safeguard in the system: If a patient ever has to explain under emergency conditions what medicine she or he is taking, the individual can do so with complete authority.

I also talk to them about the color, shape, and size of the medication as well as the substance and consequence. We've even drawn up charts to show the patient what the medicine looks like so that they'll know if they're not getting something exactly right and can phone us to help correct any error. However, with the advent and popularity of generic drugs, it makes the differentiation of medicines by color and shape more difficult.

In the case of Nardil, or phenelzine, I'm especially cautious. There's a famous legal case where a young woman entered a New York hospital emergency room and died when the medical personnel failed to realize she was being treated with Nardil for depression. They administered another drug to manage the symptoms they were witnessing, and the combination proved to be deadly. One of the most famous episodes of the TV show *Law and Order* illustrates the caution necessary when using Nardil for a patient.

42

We gave Jo Hepburn 15 milligrams of Nardil three times a day. That went on for two weeks and then we reduced the dosage drastically so she was on a maintenance level. But the drug and the dosage worked.

"It changed my whole life," she said. "I would be able to go three months without a headache. And the headaches were not as severe when I did get them. I wouldn't always go that long; maybe I could go for a month. But this was like heaven. I had entered the world again."

With that done, the mystery was finally solved.

But there is always something more the conscientious doctor feels he or she can do, and so there is an epilogue in Jo Hepburn's case.

First you have to consider her personality; she was a very firm, self-reliant, determined person. Now she would have to be on medicine for the rest of her life and that medicine would narrow considerably what she might choose to eat and drink. That didn't bother her too much; she had a great desire to end the headaches because of the way they interfered with her life, and she had a great deal of self-discipline.

But I wondered if there wasn't a way to improve her life, to reduce even further the impact that the headaches made on her.

As it happened, another way of treating migraine came along—biofeedback training. Jo Hepburn was one of those people for whom it proved very effective. We started using biofeedback at the Clinic in 1972, and this is a long-recognized adjunctive treatment of migraine.

Biofeedback training is simply a way of learning how to control, by thought and will, certain functions of the body that everybody thought couldn't be controlled at all. The rate at which the heart beats, for example, or the blood pressure level, or the temperature of the hands. How are these functions controlled?

Studies by Dr. Neal Miller of Rockefeller University have shown that by simply rewarding laboratory animals for certain responses, you could train them to increase or decrease their rate of heartbeat. In fact, the scientists went so far as to show control of the dilation of particular blood vessels by getting six of the laboratory animals to blush only in the right ear and six others to blush only in the left ear, even though these organs are supposed to controlled by sympathetic nerves.

What we really learned from that research—and much, much more—is that the autonomic nervous system is quite capable of deviating from its normal or programmed paces and learn new responses by trial and error.

With varying success, biofeedback training has been used to abort epileptic seizures, to overcome insomnia, to teach diaphragmatic breathing to asthmatic children, and to treat a patient with severe facial tics.

Biofeedback training was found to be useful in the treatment of headaches almost by accident, at the Menninger Foundation in Topeka, Kansas. The Menninger Foundation was—and continues to be—a world-renowned psychiatric hospital and research center. (In 2003, The Menninger Foundation relocated to Houston, Texas.) At Menninger, a research team under Dr. Elmer Green, head of the Menninger Psychophysiology Laboratory, was conducting research on biofeedback as a possible way of approaching certain mental and physical illnesses. The research team had gathered a group of 33 female volunteers to see if they could be taught to control certain responses, much as the laboratory animals were taught to change their heart rates.

The subjects were being tested to see if they could change the flow of blood through their limbs, specifically to increase the flow of blood to their hands. But they weren't being taught on a basis of a material reward so much has a sense of achievement. They were taught to watch meters that registered temperature. The meters were connected to sensors attached to the women's fingertips. As the flow of blood into and through their hands increased, the temperature of their hands would increase, and the needles on the meters would swing to the right to show that increase. Thus by watching the temperature of the hands, the researchers could follow the increased flow of blood through the hands—if any. These days the meters and needles have been replaced with more modern computer-generated graphs.

The women began the experiment by "thinking relaxation."

"I feel quiet . . . I am beginning to feel quite relaxed," you start out saying to yourself. "My feet feel heavy and relaxed . . . My ankles, my knees, and my hips feel heavy, relaxed, and comfortable . . . My solar plexus and the whole central portion of my body feel relaxed and quiet . . . My hands, my arms, and my shoulders feel heavy, relaxed, and comfortable . . . My neck, my jaws, and my forehead feel relaxed . . . They feel comfortable and smooth . . . My whole body feels quiet, heavy, comfortable, and relaxed."

Then the individual gradually shifts the focus of her thinking from relaxation to thinking that her hands are warm, then warmer, then hot. (See Appendix IX, Temperature Controlling Exercises.)

"I am quite relaxed . . . My arms and hands are heavy and warm . . . I feel quiet . . . My whole body is relaxed and my hands are warm, relaxed, and warm . . . My hands are warm. . . Warmth is flowing into my hands . . . They are warm . . . warmer . . . even warmer now." Some individuals think about their hands, being immersed in a bucket of increasingly hot water.

The idea is that focusing on the hands growing hot will, under biofeedback theory, increase the temperature of the hands and thereby increase the flow of blood to and through the hands.

As it happens, one day a woman who was at the moment suffering from intense migraine pain was engaged in the research. Suddenly, during one of the tests, her headache disappeared completely. Researchers quickly perceived, from the record of the instrument readings, that this happened at precisely the moment when there was a great rush of blood to her hands.

Dr. Green was sufficiently intrigued to start looking into the literature on migraine for a clue as to why this happened. He came to the feeling that cold hands were a common factor in migraine. He speculated as to whether increasing the temperature of the hands might not mean increasing the flow of blood through the hands by diverting it from the head, where it had been pulsing and throbbing through swollen and painful vessels. If that was the case, it was easy to see why the headache had disappeared: the blood flow was lessened, and thus the blood vessels were not so painfully distended.

Soon, news of the event spread through the clinic. Another migraine sufferer, the wife of one of the doctors on the staff, went to Dr. Green to see if he could help her. "I wasn't at all sure that this would work a second time," Dr. Green said. This second woman had no experience at all with biofeedback or the meters, and there was no indication that she knew or cared about the biofeedback. But Dr. Green taught her to apply the sensors and use the meters in about 15 minutes. Then he let her take a meter home so she could practice using them. She quickly learned how to make the temperature needle go up totally at will simply by thinking and focusing on the exercises. As the needle went up, the flow of blood through her hands went up, and her headache went down. "She came back two weeks later and said she was off migraine drugs completely," Dr. Green recalled. She had only one migraine episode in the next four years.

A pilot study was organized using only headache sufferers as patients, with Dr. Joseph Sargent, head of the Department of Internal Medicine at Menninger, as director of the project. Not only did the biofeedback method prove successful in reducing or eliminating headache in the vast majority of women, but 75 percent of them no longer relied on the meters within a month after starting. After training themselves with the help of the instruments, they were soon able to get along without them and raise their hand temperature, and thus the blood flow, with no external aid. It's similar to learning to ride a bicycle—once you learn it, the technique of keeping your balance seems reflexive, although it actually has taken a carefully learned system of signals to learn to keep from falling.

When I read the report of the Menninger group, I traveled to Topeka to learn this new technique and to decide whether to introduce it to my patients. I must admit that I initially had my doubts as to the utility of biofeedback, perhaps not only due to an interesting diagnostic mistake I observed during the visit. I had traveled to Topeka with two of our nurses, and we were introduced to what we were told was a migraine patient. Within about 30 seconds of meeting the patient, both the nurses and I knew that this was a cluster headache patient and not a person with migraine. His headache had the classic cluster features. Still, I decided in the affirmative, of course. There is a biofeedback room at the Clinic and an entire department at the Diamond Inpatient Unit. These rooms are kept as dark and soundproof as possible, where patients can learn biofeedback. And we've arranged for meters and sensors to be leased to our patients until they learn to use the techniques without the sensors.

We select the biofeedback patients with some care. The intangible "think your way to success" implications of the method are not within the understanding of some patients. Children, without possessing learned behavior about headaches, are most successful in learning biofeedback techniques.

"Well, I kind of doubted that this thing was going to work," Jo Hepburn admitted. "But I was willing to try anything. I think that when you're made as desperate as you are made by a migraine headache, you'll do anything to find relief. Especially if you believe in your doctor. If he believes in what he's doing, you've got to believe. And if he says it's helped people—other people—then you've got to go along with it."

She took a machine home, practiced on it conscientiously for a few days, and completely mastered the technique. She developed an individual thought technique for making her hand temperature rise.

"I've never been able to imagine that my hand was in a bucket of warm water, hot water," she said. "I imagine that I'm looking inside my hands and I can see the boiling hot blood, the boiling blood going up and down my fingers," she said. "That's how I get my hands warm. And then I get to the point where I see my hand on fire; it's that hot. I can see the flames in it. Roaring. It should be," she said with a laugh, "crisp by now."

In a few days, she was able to raise the temperature easily to a satisfactory degree. (Usually a 4-degree rise in temperature will begin having an effect on the headache.) Soon she didn't need the instruments at all; she could raise her hand temperature without them. "I think the time before last when I was in the doctor's office, I raised my [hand] temperature 24 degrees," she said. That's as much as any of our meters register.

"I only do it now when I feel that I might be getting a migraine," she said. "I know you should do it twice a day, but I don't. I just don't. I have no trouble raising the temperature of my fingers, my hands, even without practicing. I can go for weeks without practicing, but when it seems I have to do it. I can do it."

Biofeedback has given her the feeling that she, not the medicine, is in control of her life. She has the conviction that she can, at will, control her headaches and bring them to an end. She'd had only one headache in four months at the time of this writing.

"Then it came on at night. I had it when I woke up. Usually when it gets into a bad headache, and this was a bad one, biofeedback doesn't work too well. It does keep it down more. It does control it so that it doesn't get too bad; it keeps it within a certain degree. But it takes a little while to get rid of it; it doesn't just go away." That's natural enough. Because she was sleeping, she didn't have a chance to use the biofeedback training before the headache had built up its momentum. "I take zolmitriptan nasal spray If I get to that headache right at the beginning, I can control it. I've had lots of starts of headaches in the last four months, which I've gotten rid of. As long as I get rid of them, I don't count them as headaches."

In a sense, this is the ultimate course of headache treatment. It was a long time before it became effective. It took several twists and turns we didn't expect. It did not end her headaches completely, but it put her in control instead of making her the handmaiden of pain.

And it changed her life in a particular way. I tried to do it through conversations, even lectures, in the early days of treatment. I told her how she should slow down, how everything didn't have to be done in a day, how she might take some of the pressure off herself. "Don't say everything that comes into your mind." I try to explain to all my people, or that they want to be, but that they are not God and they can't do everything. They have to learn to say no once in a while in order to find out what is genuinely important to them and then to undertake projects only in those fields. It is a process of self-discovery that is useful in every walk of life.

Did my suggestions make an impact?

"No, not then," she said, "because it would have been a mark of defeat again."

"Now I can do it because I know there's a way the headaches can be controlled. And I don't have this guilt any more. That neurotic feeling. So now when I feel I'm pushing myself unnecessarily I can slow down. But then I couldn't because it was a sign of weakness. And I didn't like that. I insisted I could do everything I wanted to do."

This is not to say she's given up a somewhat frenetic life. She has written two books for children. She's in a writer's group—an organization of writers, librarians, publishers, illustrators—anyone interested in the world of books for children. She gave up women's club work. "I realized that I couldn't stand women's clubs; they just galled me," she said. She cut down on church activities. "Up until about six months ago, I did volunteer work at the retirement home. I intend to go back and do it again." She's given up her political activities. "I vote. That's it. But anything else, I don't know—that was a very enervating thing to get into. I had to admit finally that it wasn't my cup of tea. I'd rather write my beliefs down in stories, get them across that way." She does not necessarily do fewer things; she does different things.

"I finally got to the age in life where I decided that I better do the things that I can do best—that I think I can do best," she said. "Or at least that I enjoy doing, and maybe I can do them better than the things I do just because I feel I have to do them. As you can tell, my attitudes began to change. I don't know if it was because I got so much help with the headaches or what, but I began to finally readjust my life. *After* I got help with the headaches, I was finally able to see life in a different way. It wasn't such a compulsion—I didn't do thing because I felt I had to do them. I began to measure which things I could better, what ways I could make myself a better person—perhaps try and make this world a better place to live in. This may be my little corner. And in that way I would pick out what it was, instead of living each day in such complete frustration—I hated doing all these little, innocuous things that I would do simply because I felt I had to do them. I finally admitted that I didn't *have* to do anything. There are many things that I *could* do. And perhaps I *have* some talent someplace."

The curious, and human, aspect of this is that she didn't make these changes in an effort to master and manage her headaches. She made them only after she knew that she was no longer mastered by them. "It came after the headaches were pretty much gone," she said, "and not before that." In short, the sense of urgency to get things done, despite the almost crippling impact of the headaches, did not leave her until the moment she knew the headaches were only a small incident of life and not its central controlling factor. That is the one gift research has given to her and to other headache victims.

3

THE MISGUIDED MOTHER

One day a few years ago, a mother and her 13-year-old daughter came to see me about the child's chronic headaches. She had been suffering from migraine since she was eight years old, and she had been getting them about once a month. Now suddenly she was getting severe migraine almost once a day—which was a terrifying burden for anybody, and especially for a young teenager.

In talking to the mother and child about the girl's medical history, I was astonished to learn that the girl was on the Pill.

"But why?" I asked, somewhat puzzled.

"To help cure her acne," said her mother.

I decided to talk with the mother and her daughter separately. It turned out that the child thought she was on the Pill because her mother was really afraid that she, the girl, would get pregnant. There may have been some truth in this. The mother associated migraine with menstruation and when the child developed migraine at the age of eight, the mother was sure she was maturing early. So when the child had barely entered her teens, her mother persuaded the family doctor to prescribe birth control pills for the young girl. Well, the girl was advanced for her age, but this in itself is not necessarily a reflection of her being sexually active.

The girl appeared to me to be suffering from deep confusion and pervasive doubts and fears. She didn't know if her mother disapproved of her having sexual intercourse or if she simply lacked confidence in her ability, at the age of 13, to refrain from doing so. Alternatively, she wondered, did her mother really expect her to have sexual experiences and get her to take the Pill to make sure she didn't become pregnant? She simply did not accept the other reason— that she was on the Pill to cure her acne.

Obviously, the Pill alone could increase the pain and frequency of migraine. In fact, there is a one-third chance this could happen. There is also a one-third chance the headaches would stay the same, and there is a one-third chance they may actually improve. As we have seen, the Pill increases the concentration of female hormones in the body. This impact is most noticeable in women who already have shown a tendency toward migraine.

In this case, the heightened severity and the daily onset of the headache made me suspect that the girl was, in addition, suffering a very considerable stress over the unspoken sexual attitudes of her mother. And it was possible that this stress was contributing very significantly to her migraine attacks.

Fortunately, the solution wasn't hard. I recommended that the girl be taken off the Pill immediately, but I did it with a twist. I urged her mother to be the person who told the girl, as if *she* thought it best. I also encouraged the mother to speak with her daughter more openly about her maturing and the choices she will be confronting as she continues into adolescence and adulthood.

The teenager soon was free from daily migraine, though she did revert to her previous pattern of one-a-month migraine. Fortunately, there are ways to handle that problem, even in the very young, and bit by bit, she was able to manage the migraine that remained.

4

THE MISUNDERSTOOD DRUNK

Timsy Malloy was one of those inimitable characters who seemed to pass through life with a tilt as much as a lilt. He had a taste for fine liquor (well, it didn't have to be fine—just abundant) and an inclination to suffer the consequences.

He was a short, dapper man who, for a while, ran a bar and was his own bartender. He went out of business because he drank up the inventory, I fear, and he became more or less a regular patient of mine; I had him hospitalized three times for complications of the liver.

This was in the days when I was in family practice (before I concentrated on neurology and headaches) and Timsy Malloy would come in and sit in a chair in my examination room, lean forward conspiratorially, his wide, blue eyes expressing anxiety and doubt while he told me how awful he was feeling. He'd tell me about his hemorrhoids or claim that he had trouble passing water, and I'd examine him and find some more of the same old liver problem and ship him off to the hospital.

He came to me, as his "old" doctor, not too long ago complaining about a headache. Now Timsy Malloy was likely to go through life with a headache—at least with a hangover—but this one was different. He wasn't drinking because he'd been in the hospital for the past two weeks.

What happened, he said, was an accident. The way the people at the hospital saw it was that Timsy Malloy had fallen and struck his head on a curb. They suspected that he was fall-down drunk. The way that Timsy Malloy saw it was that he'd struck his head hard while getting out of his car and, what with one thing and another, he had to be carted off to the nearest emergency room with a concussion. Now when he told me that, I had to believe him, because he was never a sloppy or careless drunk; he held his liquor well, and he was very neat about his person.

In any case, he'd been out for two days and he had a headache that started in the hospital. He tried to suggest to them that hangovers don't last this long but, as is usual, they weren't terribly disturbed by his having a headache. Besides he did lurch a little when he walked, somewhat favoring his left side.

The first thing I did was put him through a neurological examination. To show you how simple it is, I asked him to put out both his hands and I tried to push down first one hand and then the other. I found it difficult to push his right hand down, but when I pressed down on this left hand, it had very little resistance.

Then I asked Timsy Malloy to squeeze my hand with one of his. Again his right hand was satisfactory, but there was a noticeable weakness when he tried to squeeze with his left hand. Next, I tested his tendon reflexes with a percussion hammer, striking appropriate spots in both his arms and his legs. In both cases, the response in his left leg and left arm was much greater than on the right side—in other words, they jumped a great deal more. He had what is called hyperactive reflexes.

He also showed a positive pathological reflex. What does that mean? Well, I stroked—tickled so to speak—the sole of his foot. Normally when you do that, the big toe will curl downward. When I did it to Timsy Malloy, the big toe on his right foot bent downward. But the big toe on his left foot bent upward, and his toes flared.

This is called a positive Babinski reflex, and it is quite significant. It usually means that there is something wrong, probably some organic disease in the brain or the spinal cord.

So I had Timsy Malloy admitted to a hospital before nightfall as an emergency case, and I quickly ordered an MRI (Magnetic Resonance Imaging). This is simply a way of getting an image of something in or around the brain—whether it is a tumor or a blood clot or a problem in the blood vessels of the

54

head—that may be causing problems. A computerized axial tomography (CT) scan may also be used to diagnose a subdural hematoma, but an MRI can disclose some cases that the CT will miss. In this particular case, it showed us that Timsy Malloy had a large blood clot under the lining that surrounds the brain.

Undoubtedly, he had ruptured some of the blood vessels in this lining when he bumped his head, and a clot had formed in the area. The danger in a clot of this kind is that it gets larger and larger and brings pressure on the brain. It gets larger because it acts like a sponge and absorbs serum and other fluids from the region around it. Because it is in an entirely closed space, it cannot expand endlessly. It puts pressure on the brain, and causes increasingly complex and distressing problems.

Once we spotted the clot and accurately located it, we ordered surgery. It is not a terribly difficult surgical procedure. It is a matter of drawing off the material in the clot. But it is a delicate procedure. Fortunately, in Timsy Malloy's case, the surgeon cleaned it up quickly and completely, and when everything was over, he felt no pain, and he was soon back to his old drinking habits. With mild subdural hematomas, a course of steroids may be sufficient to resolve the problem, but this was not the case with Timsy Malloy.

5

THE PAINFUL HAT

One autumn day not too long ago, an elderly man, some 68 years old, came to me with a most peculiar problem: he got terrible pains in his head when he wore a hat. With winter coming, this was, naturally, a source of some concern to him. But it is not the type of problem that normally sends a person running to a headache specialist. However, he was beginning to have pain even when he wasn't wearing a hat. It was intense when he did something as simple as chew his food; often he couldn't finish eating because of the intense stabbing pain in his head. It had reached a point where it hurt even when he opened his mouth.

"I can't sleep much at night," he grumbled. Because he tended to sleep with his mouth open, he felt a terrible pain in his head.

He had a number of other complaints, principally about muscle pain and pain in the neck, hips, and general body area. To many people, these might sound like the complaints of an older man—but it turned out they were important clues to the cause of his head pain.

We gave him our customary in-office physical and neurological exams. He tested negative in both areas, but we did see some tiny red nodules on the painful side of his head, around the temple. This was where he said the pain was worse. His hatband would, I could see, press on both sides of his head, but he said it was a more intense stabbing sensation on the right side than on the left.

I ran my fingers over the temporal artery on the right side. That's the artery in the temple where a pulse can often be felt. But when I felt and even pressed on this artery gently, I didn't feel a pulse. It wasn't that he didn't have one, rather, the artery did not feel flexible, as do normal arteries. It felt hard, almost like a piece of string under the skin of his temple. By now I was convinced that this man was suffering a headache pain that fell into the "traction" or "inflammatory" category; that is to say, it had an organic origin.

57

I thought I had some pretty good clues as to the probable cause. From immediate examination, there were two types of attack that it might be. One is called tic douloureux (trigeminal neuralgia). It may be felt in any part of the face but rarely below the lower jawbone. The pain is of a jabbing, even burning quality. It may occur spontaneously, but more likely it is initiated by cold air or a light touch on the skin of the cheek—or by biting, chewing, yawning, swallowing—even sneezing or talking. The pain is usually described as a high-intensity "jab" that lasts for 20 to 30 seconds. Then it stops for up to a minute before the victim gets another jab of pain. This on-again-off-again pain can go on for an hour at a time.

The other is called temporal arteritis (the itis in any medical term means "inflammation"); so the terms, temporal arteritis means "inflammation of the artery in the temple." When these arteries become inflamed, it hurts to touch them—even the touch of a hatband can cause pain. And with it, one finds, for some curious reason, an accompanying pain in other points, just as this patient had described. One thing I knew: a decision had to be made quickly as to which of these two possible causes was the correct one. For one of the somber effects of temporal arteritis is that if it's not caught early, it may lead to blindness.

One thing that can be done rather readily is to confirm the presence of inflammation and, by that, the presence of temporal arteritis. This is done through what is called a sedimentation test. We put some red blood cells from the patient into a serum and wait to see how long it takes for the sediment—called the erythrocyte—to settle out of the serum. If it takes an unusually long time—more than an hour for anything up to 15 millimeters for a man—then we believe that inflammation is present. In this case, the rate was three times as long as normal. That was enough to make us feel strongly that the problem was temporal arteritis. But to confirm this diagnosis, there was yet another step, and it reflects some of the subtle dimensions of medicine. Temporal arteritis was described first in 1890, and further insights were offered in 1932 and 1968. But a thousand years ago, in a book called *Tabkivat al Kahhalin*, an Arabic medical primer, there was a suggestion of what we now call a biopsy for certain chronic diseases, including one involving a sharp biting inflammation of the arteries of the temple where loss of vision was a common aftermath.

Today, a biopsy is merely a common and effective way of confirming the disease. We had the patient admitted to the hospital quickly for a simple biopsy, (though many of these procedures are now done on an outpatient basis). The biopsy is done with a local anesthetic, without any particular discomfort to the patient. The tissue is then examined by a pathologist, who confirms or rejects the presence of the disease. In this case, a definite diagnosis of temporal arteritis was confirmed.

But in that ancient Arabian medical primer, it was suggested that biopsy in itself had a curative effect, and that was confirmed in 1968 by some experiments in Germany. Just why—well, we don't quite know. In this particular case I wasn't inclined to rely entirely on the biopsy. I went to a more classical treatment involving steroids, the most common of which is prednisone. We watched the patient closely to determine whether there were any signs of blindness; fortunately, there were not. But we continued him on steroids for six months. You cannot wisely maintain a patient endlessly on steroids, and so we knew we wanted the disease conquered within that time.

On his last visit to us, I knew we'd done it. As I entered the examination room, he winked and nodded toward a coat tree in a corner. There, hanging on it, was the symbol of his freedom from pain—the hat that he'd been wearing.

6

THE MIXED PAIN

The letter gave only a hint of the pain. "For more than 10 years," it read, "I've suffered recurring, persistent, daily headaches. . . . The problem has worsened to the point that now, at age 24, I cannot hold a job or otherwise engage in normal activities of daily living. I've been totally disabled by headaches—some spells are severe enough that I cannot get out of bed for several days.... I'm unable to make any definite plans for tomorrow or next week because the headaches come sporadically—some days worse than others, some days totally crippling, other days tolerable. I must have immediate attention. . . . Please consider this an *urgent* plea, for I no longer have the strength or ability to cope with this problem. . . ."

Another warning—more than a plea—came a few days before her appointment. Terry Patterson lived in central Ohio and was flying to Chicago to our Headache Clinic. But she was obviously so distraught in making the airline reservation that the airline people checked with me.

"What do you recommend, Doctor?" asked the airline agent, a trace of agitation seasoning her otherwise cool and impersonal voice, "if your patient collapses on the plane?" Collapses! Here I hadn't even seen the patient and outside parties were warning me of her collapse.

When I met Terry Patterson, I began to understand why. Once she'd been a vital, personable girl, with dates every weekend—every weekend that was possible—good grades in school and an abundance of fulfilling activities. Now, in her mid-20s, she was a gray, blurred mass. She was overweight (180 pounds on her first visit), with an oddly stiff posture and glasses whose lenses seemed mismatched. She had, as I came to know, a mind that was quick and understanding, but she rarely offered her opinion. Her defenses were too high.

61

For she lived almost half her life with a pain that she couldn't escape and that no one could treat.

The patient I saw before me was in the agony of headache pain and in a state of total disintegration. This is one of the notable and most dismaying characteristics of chronic headache. We can see its effects in the quiet crumbling of an otherwise normal individual, very much as we might see the quicker disabling effects of a stroke or a tumor or a catastrophic heart attack.

At first we think—the patient thinks, his or her family thinks—that recovery is possible, or even likely, as a headache ends. But then as it strikes again and again and again, we come to know that the disintegration is real, but slower, if ever laced with the false hope that the pain is finally over.

It is not only the pain but the inevitability of pain—the knowledge that there is no end to it short of self-destruction—that attacks the psyche and ruins the human personality.

Terry Patterson was sure she had migraine. She was right, she *did* have migraine, but she had something more, and it never dawned on the 10 or 12 doctors who had treated her to look for a particular something more. She was bright enough to offer the barest suggestion that more than one kind of pain was plaguing her. But the responsibility for failing to find the reason why must lie, I feel, with the practitioner of medicine. For headache victims usually don't know that there is more than one kind of headache bothering them. Then they get a pain in the head, they figure it's migraine or a brain tumor. But as we've seen, there are many, many causes of headache pain—and many more than you are yet to learn about—and it's up to the doctor to discern these causes and to treat the pain. Multiple cases of headache are not that unusual in modern medicine, and it was not difficult to start attacking the pain they were causing for Terry Patterson. The real tragedy was in her futile search for relief and in the complete frustration of her failure.

She was 13 when the headaches first became bothersome. "I'd come home with a splitting headache," she remembered, "have to go to bed, take two aspirin, sleep two or three hours." She went to the family doctor several times as the headaches got worse, and his prescription was, she recalled, "Don't worry. Don't be concerned. These things are normal for someone your age."

Years later she was still disgusted, perhaps embittered, that the doctor did not even recommend eye tests (her eyes were bad, but nobody knew it) or metabolism tests (perhaps to explain why she was then overweight).

As she progressed through high school, the headaches became worse. They focused behind her right eye, but they seemed to affect her whole head. "Headaches were deep inside my head," she said, "and the only relief was to lie down and close my eyes." Her eyes were constantly tired, even burning. "I felt like something was pulling at the back of my eyes." She felt, in some moments of migraine, "empty headed," as if her "head felt hungry."

Nevertheless, she maintained an A average in high school, and she was busy in social events, on school committees, in sports. In short, she was showing some of the compulsion for achievement—despite pain—that we so often see in migraine victims.

The summer after she graduated from high school, she went to an eye specialist. He prescribed glasses for nearsightedness and, although she wore the glasses only part-time, the headaches went away for the rest of the summer.

In the autumn, she started as a freshman at Ohio State, intending to become a teacher, and the headaches came back—slowly, insinuatingly. She took over-the-counter headache remedies and tried to sleep the pain away. "But in those days, I never awoke without one or went to school without knowing or being afraid I'd get one," she said. She was busy and happy with her schoolwork. But she often felt terribly fatigued, and she was frustrated by the way the headaches interfered with the pace she wanted to set in school, particularly as they began increasing in severity and frequency.

Sometime after her sophomore year, she went to another eye specialist. He changed her prescription in her lenses but didn't remark on anything else wrong with her eyes. She continued to wear the glasses only part-time. In any case, the change in the spectacles again seemed to help end the headaches—for a couple of weeks.

But they returned gradually, and they seemed worse. "Often the headaches came at midday and I was so exhausted—I felt like I was starving and I'd eat candy or an ice cream bar to lessen the headache so I could finish the school day." (Interestingly, she used an infusion of blood sugar from the sweets because she had discovered, by trial and error, that it seemed to reduce the headache.) The link between migraine and obesity is an area of increasing interest, with the latest data suggesting a greater prevalence of obesity in chronic migraine patients. More research needs to be conducted to assess whether significant weight loss will help to improve patients' headaches, but most headache specialists agree that moderate exercise tends to be helpful.

Next, she went to a gynecologist, who ordered a thyroid profile. "I was put on thyroid hormone replacement immediately," she said. "I gradually noticed a great difference. The terrible fatigue was gone. I was active more hours a day, and I was happy about this." But now she was *expecting* the headache to strike. "The headaches came about noon almost daily, but if I took two Excedrin, or more, if necessary, I could usually finish a day's plans. The times I was really sick with headaches which Excedrin would not help were the few days following or preceding my menstrual period. My eyes burned, my head burned, pinched, and ached each time, and I'd have to take several Excedrin— four to six—to combat cramps and headache and to get through a day." Here is the first clue that the daily headaches were different from the menstrual (or, in her case, migraine) headaches; the over-the-counter remedy could reach one but not always the other.

Halfway through her junior year, she took the first step toward surrender. You don't know how hard this is for the driver and the doer. But you've got to remember that she had had these headaches for six-and-a-half years and nothing had brought them to a permanent end. Indeed, they seemed to get worse. "I was discouraged about my health and the limitations it placed on me," she reported. "I needed time away from school to think. I was tired of everything—school, fighting what was becoming a daily headache problem. I stayed out of school in the spring, worked part-time in the family business, slept a lot, went to a couple of evening meetings a week, and was active in a limited sense but only several hours a day."

She also began a round of seeing doctors that lasted for more than 18 months. She went back to the eye specialist, and he discovered a condition called aniseikonia, in which the size and shape that one eye casts on the retina differs from that cast upon its retina by the other eye. This would explain the burning and fatigue of her eyes during high school years—something unrelieved by her earlier eyeglasses. Now she began to wear glasses with different lenses all the time.

Then she went to an eye, ear, nose, and throat specialist in the belief that her headaches might be sinus-oriented. He told her no. She went to another doctor to see about a lump in her throat. She thought perhaps this reflected an allergy or perhaps a sinus condition which was causing the headaches. He told her the lump in her throat was "probably a swollen lymph node—nothing to worry about."

She decided—after an 18-month "sabbatical"—to go back to Ohio State. She lived with some cousins near campus, took five courses, was determinedly active, "yet needed Excedrin and naps daily to keep going." The headaches remained with her, but she still had hope of getting help for them; after all, she'd only been to six doctors so far.

So, she went to an endocrinologist, who ran a number of tests and found nothing. "She said my headaches were due to my being nervous about my future. I *was* nervous about my future, with student teaching coming up!" In any case, the endocrinologist took her off thyroid ("which had helped me so much") and prescribed for her what she calls "three-a-day nerve tablets to take if I felt a headache coming on." The nerve tablets helped "for a week or so," she said. And then she went back to taking Excedrin to get through the day.

65

The pressure on her began to build up. She went into student teaching, and she kept fighting the "splitting" headaches. "I was exhausted by noon," she said. She took the "nerve" medicine and the Excedrin, and she felt herself sliding toward helplessness. At first, she thought she'd have to quit school because of the pressure, although she was very close to graduation. She went back to the endocrinologist, who, Terry remembered a trifle bitterly, "said she couldn't help me." At that point, she felt she was going to have a nervous breakdown. "I lost hope of finding help."

She didn't break down altogether. She would come much closer to that in the future. But now she struggled through to graduation, building a cumulative grade-point average of 3.2 (4.0 points would be straight A). That was a remarkable and characteristic feat, considering how deeply troubled she was by her headache pain.

But after graduation she didn't have any drive left. "I didn't know what to do or where to turn. I stayed home, helped in the family business—could make no plans, would make no plans." She tried volunteering in several work areas, such as Sunday school tutoring, but was gulping down Excedrin to do it. It was the price she had to pay for any accomplishment, however, small.

"This became the firmly established pattern of my life: for every day or evening spent in an activity, I'd have to spend hours in bed, recovering—using ice packs, massagers, heating pads, and Excedrin to reduce the pounding pain in time for the next project. If I didn't get those rest periods, if I kept pushing beyond, then the pain got so severe I'd have to spend days in bed."

Time was like an accordion for her. There would be a few moments of expansive highs, where there was no pain; then a squeezing, almost crushing blow when the pain returned. Ultimately, she went to a neurosurgeon, who gave her a neurological examination—negative. He ordered an MRI—negative. He ordered another EEG - also negative. After another serious episode, in which she collapsed from pain while visiting a girlfriend on a long weekend, she went back to the neurosurgeon. "He told me I might have to live this way all my life. He

66

said if I had a positive attitude, I could do anything I wanted." But she wanted to get rid of the headaches, and a positive attitude had no effect on them.

Nevertheless, he gave her some medicine. "Gray pills." They worked for a while. "Stopped the pinching in the back of the neck completely but not the frontal headaches, pulling over the eyes, and all that." Here was the second clue that she knew there were two different locations of pain—one in the back of her neck and the other in the front of her head—and that the medicine attacked one locale but not the other. Just that awareness might have alerted the neurologist to the possibility that she was suffering from two different kinds of headache.

In the meantime, she decided on another course of action. She decided that she'd change her entire lifestyle, move across the country, and try to escape the pain. She had grown up in an industrial environment, but she loved the outdoors, and so she applied for a job with the National Park Service and got one at Sequoia National Park in California.

I liked my job and I loved the park," said Terry Patterson. She was wary about the headaches continuing, but she was sure, in this environment, she could cope with them. She was wrong. As time passed in her first summer there, the headaches didn't diminish, they became "more devastating" and more frequent. Soon she felt, as she had in college, cut off from all she wanted by the pain in her head. "I became depressed much of the time because often I couldn't talk to or be with my friends because of this."

Sequoia is a region of spectacular redwoods, towering granite peaks, deep canyons, and alpine lakes. It removes a person in time and spirit from a wretched past but not from a tormenting present. "The headaches continued to mount," she confessed, "as the weeks passed, forcing me to spend hours in bed after work each day. By the last month or so, I wasn't conscious of anything else around me—only the headaches. The only way I can think to describe it is I was split between my misery and the people around me. For weeks afterward, I had to fight constant fear and depression after going through this experience."

She lost interest in being outdoors. She couldn't think of anything to say to friends. She'd take 9 to 12 Excedrin a day just to combat the threat of headaches. She suffered a hot, stuffy, prickly feeling in the head when she didn't suffer outright pain. She admits she was "so highly emotional, I don't know what it feels like to see things normally or in perspective."

Excedrin contains caffeine and, as we have discussed previously, caffeine can help headache due to its vasoconstrictive properties. Too much caffeine, however, can not only cause a headache condition to worsen, but as Terry Patterson experienced, excessive caffeine can lead to even more problems such as insomnia and worsening anxiety.

In the past during her menstrual period, she'd suffered headaches in which the pounding in her head was so bad that she told friends that everything in the room seemed to "echo" to it. She felt then that her head would "explode," and for several days afterward the temples of her skull were sore to the touch. Now she began getting the same kind of headaches, during her periods, at Sequoia. "Without Excedrin, the headaches became so severe that I couldn't see, and I had to leave work at noon. With Excedrin, pain was bearable for a few hours, but the pressure increased, requiring hours of extra rest."

Eventually she knew that her attempt to flee pain had failed. She decided to go back to Ohio.

"I came home completely irrational in thinking and talking," she said. "I couldn't sleep regularly for weeks. I felt as if I had a split personality from the mounting headaches and quantities of Excedrin the last month at Sequoia. It was weeks before I saw friends or could talk to them. I was afraid I was insane at times."

At home, the pain cycle continued and she became more and more despondent. She couldn't take a job because she was afraid she'd have to be in bed for three or four days a week. "It seems that everything results in a headache. They come daily regardless of what I do—sleep too much or too little, exercise too much or too little, laugh or cry or get excited. There's no pattern apparent to me, other than that it is an unbearable pattern in which I am restricted from working or from living a normal life. "Eventually," she said, "the headaches seemed to last 24 hours a day." She was gulping 13 to 15 Excedrin a day—"then I couldn't hold anything in my stomach." Headache remedies couldn't help her, doctors couldn't help her. In fact, nothing it seemed could help her. "I wondered whether it was worthwhile going on living," she said.

One January day the winter after she left Sequoia, she read about headache specialists and the work I was doing at the Headache Clinic. That's when we got the letter and the phone call from the airline.

It was clear, by the time she arrived at our office, that she was very emotionally upset. But that was no reason not to treat her or to dismiss her problem by suggesting the pain was all in her mind or by saying, "You'll just have to live with it." Clearly the pain was so great and constant that she *couldn't* live with it, and that was what caused the emotional disturbance. I'd venture that almost anybody would be emotionally upset if they'd spent almost half a lifetime looking forward every day to nothing but unbearable and inescapable pain.

There was no mystery about her emotional problem. She was in long-term clinical depression. I don't mean the kind of "I'm feeling blue" depression that strikes all of us at one time or another and then disappears in a few hours or a day. I'm talking about the long-term depression that lasts for a year or two—or even six to eight years. Indeed, the depression settles so permanently on the patient that sometimes he doesn't know he has a depression; he thinks life is always lived that way.

Similarly, there was no mystery about her pain. She had a very severe migraine, of course. The pain within her head and in the temple and frontal lobes was characteristic of migraine. The timing—with her menstrual period—was characteristic of migraine. Her compulsive personal drive, until gradually defeated, was also characteristic of migraine. But she also had another kind of headache—actually she was suffering from two different kinds of chronic

69

recurrent headache pain and daily pain. The latter was the headache that caused pain in the back of her neck—the pinched feeling. It was a condition which was interrupting her sleep and interfering with her ability to concentrate. She was, in short, suffering from depression. And why not? If you'd spent all those years wondering, not if, but when during the day you were going to suffer Draconian pain, you would fall in to a depression also. Depression had helped precipitate her transformation to chronic migraine.

Chronic Migraine is defined as 15 or more headache days per month, and when a patient's headache condition progresses from the occasional headache to one with this frequency, the term used among headache specialists is "transformation." The headache *transforms* from the occasional severe headache that tends to occur only a few times per month, after which the patient returns to her normal baseline of no headache, into what may seem like an altogether different condition, one in which the severe headache days continue to occur, but the return to normal baseline of no headache is no longer a reality for the patient. Complete recovery between attacks is often replaced by a lower-level headache or incomplete migraine recovery. Many patients with chronic migraine do, in fact, suffer from headache every single day.

We used to think that patients suffered from either migraine or tension-type headache, and that they rarely were considered to have both. As we have learned more about migraine, however, we have better understood that a patient with migraine, especially chronic migraine, can have some headaches with more of the traditional "migraine" features, such as nausea, photophobia, and phonophobia as well as other headaches with more typical "tension" features, such as a hatband-like distribution of pain about the head with or without neck pain. These days headache specialists tend to include both of these headaches under the "umbrella" of migraine.

There are certain conditions that increase the likelihood that a patient's migraine will transform from episodic to chronic. Anxiety and depression are the most common conditions the can lead to transformation. Nearly half of all chronic migraine patients suffer from either anxiety or depression, or both. The nature of both anxiety and depression is that they both can lead to interrupted sleep—typically the anxious person has difficulty falling asleep, while the depressed person may wake often throughout the night. Interrupted sleep can be a headache trigger for a great many migraine patients. Sleep is not the only mechanism by which these psychiatric conditions can play a role in the transformation to chronic migraine.

The degree to which I personally feel that depression can play a role in chronic migraine is perhaps best illustrated when one considers how I started my career in headache. I presented an exhibit at the 1961 American Medical Association meeting entitled, "The Masks of Depression." I observed that physical symptoms, including headache, were, in fact, "masks" that suggested underlying depression in patients. At that meeting, one of the few doctors in the country treating headache, Lester Blumenthal, who would later become a good friend, asked if I had ever treated headache patients with tricyclic antidepressants. This intrigued me and lay the foundation for my pursuit of research into the use of tricyclic antidepressants in migraine. After meeting Dr. Blumenthal, I would also present my findings to the American Academy for the Study of Headache (AASH), which later became the American Headache Society.

As I talked with Terry Patterson, I had to consider the choices in treatment available to me. She was clearly suffering from chronic migraine, as her headache had transformed from an episodic condition to a constant one. Given her excessive use of Excedrin, she also suffered from medication overuse headache, in which the frequent use of a medication used to treat headache can actually cause an increase in headache over time. She needed to be admitted to the Diamond Headache Inpatient Unit at Presence St. Joseph Hospital. She was willing to do whatever was necessary to get her back to the job she loved at Sequoia, so she agreed to be admitted.

I explained to Terry Patterson that during her stay in the unit we would have five goals to accomplish, and that each goal was as important as the next. I emphasized that the goals were geared toward her having improved function over the long-term rather than just when she left the hospital. The first goal was to break the headache cycle, that everyday headache that had become constant, with more severe hours and days mixed in. At best, her headache had only returned to the baseline moderate pain level. If we were able to break the headache cycle, she could look forward to having fewer episodes of severe headache and even some days without any headache pain. We would use a variety of intravenous medications to accomplish this goal, but the primary medication we would use is the vasoconstrictor dihydroergotamine (DHE). She would receive nine doses of DHE over the course of three days. I warned her that she may experience nausea with the medication but assured her that we would help her to manage this symptom. She agreed that if the headache improved, she was willing to feel at least a little bit nauseated.

The second goal of the inpatient program is to start prevention medication to help lessen the frequency and severity of migraine. In Terry Patterson's case, I prescribed an antidepressant, amitriptyline. I explained to her that this medication would take three to four weeks to begin working on reducing the frequency and severity of her headaches. Since she was also suffering from depression, this was a particularly appropriate choice. The sedating effect of amitriptyline could also help her to sleep at night.

I explained to her that the third goal was to use various IV medications not only to lessen the pain that she was experiencing while she was in the inpatient unit, but also to identify which medications would be most helpful to send with her once she was discharged home. Often, if a patient responds particularly well to one of these IV medications, I can choose an oral or intramuscular version of the medication to be used at home. I explain to patients, as I did in this case, that I want them to have a virtual "toolbox" of options to treat their headaches when they occur.

72

The fourth goal of the inpatient unit is to use nondrug treatments to improve patients' headaches. These include biofeedback, which we have described earlier, acupuncture, an individual psychological assessment, and various classes geared toward assisting the patient to have a better understanding not only of her headache condition but of the various medications used to help treat that condition. Although some patients can be hesitant to embrace this particular goal, it is nevertheless a crucial part of the treatment and eventual improvement of our patients.

In Terry Patterson's case there was a fifth goal. Since she was also suffering from the overuse of Excedrin, the fifth goal was to help her to stop taking Excedrin. This goal was possibly the most important goal in her case, because if she were to continue to take Excedrin in this frequency, the other interventions would be much less likely to work. Her motivation to return to work made her an ideal candidate to accomplish this and the other goals.

"When can we start?" She asked with enthusiasm. I admitted her to the inpatient unit the same day and she began treatment with DHE later that evening. While she did experience some mild nausea with the infusion, she reported to me the next morning during rounds that this nausea was tolerable. "Like I said, anything to get me back to Sequoia!" she said emphatically. She would continue DHE every eight hours for a total of nine doses. I visited her every morning in the hospital. These days it is somewhat rare for patients to see their primary physicians if they are admitted to the hospital, but they instead are seen by hospitalists, physicians who specialize in hospital medicine. While this may be effective for a general medical patient, in the case of headache patients we strongly feel that the primary headache specialist who is working with the patient in the office should also see the patient while he or she is admitted to the hospital. Patients strongly prefer this as well.

Terry Patterson was initially hesitant to try biofeedback. When we discussed it in the office before her admission, she admitted to her skepticism that it would help her and her headache. Once the technician explained further

73

and demonstrated the use of the equipment, She felt more comfortable with the concept. When we reviewed her biofeedback reports during morning rounds throughout her hospital stay, I noticed that she became quite adept at reducing the tension in the muscles of her forehead during the sessions. She also was able to increase the temperature of her finger consistently throughout the sessions. "I didn't realize I would be able to control my tension so well. I guess I'm more powerful than I thought!" she said. I encouraged her to practice biofeedback every day, and to incorporate it into her approach to headaches when they occur.

During the inpatient stay, we identified that diphenhydramine (Benadryl) and orphenadrine (Norflex) were helpful at reducing her headache. The only side effect she reported was mild sedation with Benadryl. We agreed that, upon discharge, Terry Patterson would have a tablet version of orphenadrine as part of her toolbelt of medications to treat her headache since it was helpful in the IV form.

In addition to biofeedback she participated in classes and workshops each day during her stay at the Diamond Inpatient Unit, including a pharmacy class to learn about the various medications we use to treat headache. She met with a psychologist and agreed to follow up on referrals given to her to see a psychologist at home.

When I saw Terry Patterson on the fifth morning of her hospital stay, I opened her door and she exclaimed, "It worked! My headache is gone! I can't believe it!" Although I shared in her excitement at her current absence of headache, I assured her that in all likelihood her headache would return at some point, but probably at a much less severe level than before. We reviewed the medications with which she would go home and I emphasized that she should call the office if she has any questions. She also agreed to schedule an appointment with a psychologist.

She came back for her follow-up visit the next month, and she was so exhilarated over the decline of headache pain that now she was making many plans. Could she go back to Sequoia National Park, she asked. On the one hand, she wanted terribly to return and work there when she wasn't plagued by headaches. On the other hand, she was apprehensive about being so far away from the Headache Clinic for a prolonged period.

The first instinct was to worry about her returning to a place of failure. She'd had such a miserable experience there the previous summer that there was always the danger that remembered times and remembered place, always of terrible pain, would throw her back into depression. But the whole point of our treatment is to bring our patients back to a level of activity and interest where they can function normally in life. That means reducing the pain which has cut them off from life.

If Terry Patterson wanted to go to Sequoia, she was signaling that she felt able to cope with life again. I urged her to go back. Well, she went to Sequoia and she had a marvelous time.

Because of her trip west, it was seven months before I saw her in Chicago again. She was better than ever. She was still getting headaches, but they were only a fraction of what they had been. She was still concerned about her physical condition—there was a throbbing in a mass overlying the left carotid artery which she'd first noticed five years earlier—and I felt we might take a look into that in the near future. (As it turned out, it was more annoying than critical.) I took her pulse—it was a little high—and I changed her medication slightly and told her to come back in a month. When she did, she reported the reduction in headache pain was greater than ever.

So, she continued to come once a month, then once every two months, then every six to eight months. Bit by bit, we managed to get the migraine headache under control. It is not completely gone; perhaps it never will be. But it has been greatly lessened. She knows now that something can be done to control it—and that something is faithful adherence to her prescribed medication. The important thing is that she is no longer tyrannized by headache; she is no longer driven to the edge of despair by its pain. She is free to live her life as she envisioned it. She has conquered the pain; it has not conquered her.

"I feel," she says simply, "as if I've been reborn."

7

THE UNMOTIVATED MAYOR

He had the bulk of "The Boss". His massive head was set on his shoulders so that it seemed to turn like a tank turret, and his heavy-fingered hands seemed suited to a Dutch sailor. A variety of small craters roughened his face so that it looked as if it had suffered a miniature barrage. He was the mayor of a small Midwestern community, and he was one of the most successful in the business. He'd taken that community from a formless, little rural crossroads and made it into a thriving, prosperous, beautifully disciplined organism.

The trouble that had brought him to me was a severe and recurring headache. It didn't settle at any one place, it didn't come at any one time. It hadn't left him incapacitated as yet, but it was interfering with his work. Once it hit, he couldn't concentrate on his work, or continue it.

As we sat and talked, I could see certain elements in his physical makeup. He had a strong, square chin. He'd apparently had acne when he was younger—from the scars on his face—and we often associate acne with somewhat oily skin. But his skin was curiously dry and tough.

He had other complaints besides the headache. He was gaining weight. He'd gained 43 pounds in the last few months and he was losing interest in his life and his work. He said he recently felt tired and unable to cope with his civic duties, he had avoided city council meetings, and he no longer plunged into party politics with the zest that had made him so powerful. He said he was not interested in facing the day—or the night. He complained that he seemed to have lost his sex drive. In all this there were clues. Were the pains due to cluster headaches? There was some evidence of this; the square chin and the tough-textured, pocked skin are often seen in patients with cluster headaches. Moreover, these headaches will strike men in their 40s; unlike migraine, they are not headaches that tend to strike in the younger years and fade out in the middle

77

years. But the pattern of pain was completely unlike cluster headache. The clusters usually come in groups of two, three, four, or more a day. They tend to come to the same spot in the head and they tend to recur about the same time the next day; but this wasn't true in the mayor's case.

Were the headache pains due to depression? The general malaise he felt is often associated with depression—the reluctance to get up and face the day, the loss of zest for living, the general feeling of fatigue. But patients locked in depression don't often gain that much weight in that short a time. And he had not articulated in the course of our remarkably frank and open discussion, any reason why he might feel depressed. Was the pain due to some organic difficulty? Well, the only way we'd find out was to examine him.

There was no indication of trouble in his physical test. There was no indication of trouble in his neurological test. But there's another test we find important to administer to a good many patients, and that's a thyroid test. There were certain clues in his appearance and complaints that made me think "thyroid"; one of them was his dry and tough skin, another was his rapid weight gain, and still another was his general feeling of lassitude.

The thyroid gland is situated on the windpipe below the Adam's apple. Among other things it secretes thyroxin which seems to regulate the pace at which the body functions. When too much is secreted, the body roars through its daily activities like a thoroughbred heading down the stretch. When too little thyroxin is secreted, the individual begins to behave like a bear in hibernation. That person will feel tired, lack drive, and is more inclined to go to bed and sleep it through than to get up and attack the problems of the day. In short, he or she feels very much like the mayor did. Except the mayor had a headache to go with it.

So we gave him, in the office, thyroid tests that measure the quantity and the rate of different thyroid secretions (T-3 and T04 tests). They showed decisively that the mayor's thyroid gland was not functioning properly; indeed, it was very deficient in secreting thyroxin. This type of thyroid problem is easily treated. We put the mayor on a medication that provided the needed substances at a normal rate.

The answer was as simple as that. In a gratifyingly short time, he began losing weight—he dropped 40 pounds in a few months. He became motivated and aggressive once again and was filled with the heady exhilaration of life and power. He threw himself into his civic and political work with an irrepressible enthusiasm.

And then a year after we last saw him, he came back to the office, again bothered by headaches, again filled with indifference to his life and his work, and again gaining weight. What had gone wrong?

It was absurdly simple. He'd run out of his medication six months after his last visit, and he couldn't get it refilled automatically. We have a rule in our office that everything we prescribe is nonrefillable after six months (and some of it is nonrefillable sooner than that). The rule holds for drugs which we know to be absolutely safe as well as for those about which there are continuing questions. The reason is that some people will go on taking a medicine for a year or longer without going back to the doctor to check out whether the dosages or prescription should be changed.

If patients can't refill their prescriptions after six months, and if they feel any discomfort, then they can make another appointment so we can see how they're doing.

It is better to examine a patient to determine what, if anything, needs to be changed in his treatment than to let him go on mindlessly year after year taking a medicine he may not need. It is better to be able to take him off medication altogether when and if it's possible. And in many cases it is possible. In headaches linked to depressive or anxiety conditions, we might wean the patient off his drugs after long therapy and careful observation. In certain migraine pain, not infrequently, we can shift a patient from taking drugs daily to taking drugs only when he or she feels the migraine coming on. (Or, by using biofeedback, we can sometimes leave either the migraine patient or the depression—anxiety type headache patient free of pain and of drugs altogether.) This is not to say there is anything wrong in taking proper drugs for proper purposes; there is no more stigma in having to take medicine for headache pain than in having to take insulin for diabetes. But becoming pain-free and drug-free at the same time is not achieved by neglect or indifference on the part of the patient or on the part of the doctor. It is achieved only by an awareness by both patient and doctor of the link between, and the implications of, the illness and its treatment. And that can be achieved only by a continuing close relationship between patient and doctor.

For example, the mayor's low thyroid condition didn't disappear just because his medicine ran out. It is a continuing condition that needs to be supervised. But he was too busy in his renewed zest for this work to come back and see us, even when we phoned and asked, then insisted he come see us, or any other doctor. He kept putting if off again and again until he was sinking again into his low thyroid state—at which time he had to fight his fatigue just to make a visit. But he got his headache again, and that pain motivated him to return. We just made another examination; it had, after all, been well over a year since the last one. We found pretty much the same condition. We prescribed the same medicine, told him it was not refillable after six months, and told him why.

"So come back and see us in six months," I suggested. "We get along, we have good conversations, we have a nice relationship as two men in the professions—so why not continue it?" And, implicit in all this, why not avoid these episodes of headache and lassitude altogether?

He agreed, and his agreement helped end the headaches and his other problems. He realized he had to grant his health the same kind of discipline that he gave to politics.

8

THE SMOTHERED SYMPTOMS

The flight attendant who came to see me one afternoon a few years ago was a vital young woman filled with a spontaneous Gaelic charm.

She had been a flight attendant until she got married three or four months earlier, and she had clearly brought as much joy to the job as she got out of it. Indeed, she'd just gone back on the flight list, largely, she said, because she found the work so rewarding. On first meeting her, there was no hint of an anxiety or sense of insecurities in her relationship. She was, quite the contrary, full of independent sureness and aware of scrutiny with other people. She gave the impression that she had always enjoyed a quality of love and a love of quality, first, within her family, then in the world around her. Perhaps that is not always a good thing, for people who have always been loved have that terrible confidence that the world is going to allow them to fulfill themselves.

But she had a flaw that separated her from fulfillment. She had a chronic and recurring headache. It was not a simple headache, the pain was all over her head, not just on one side or the other. It was not an occasional pain; it came quite often, virtually every day, and it was unrelenting—it lasted much of the day. She'd returned to her job because she got so much satisfaction from it, and because she thought the variety and busyness of the work might help her overcome the headaches. Now she realized her work had not interrupted the headaches; her headaches interfered with her work.

From the in-office physical, the headache didn't seem to be organic in origin. From the interview and case history, it did not seem to be migraine, there was no history of headache in the family, it never focused on one side, there was no nausea, no vomiting, no aura. Yet she had a headache almost every day—a tight, pinched feeling around the head and neck, and general pains throughout the head.

The most obvious alternative—from the timing and locale of the headache—was that it was a chronic tension-type headache due to deep depression or severe anxiety. Yet she displayed none of the more obvious and superficial of either. There were no psychic symptoms. Her work, when she was feeling well, had not really slowed down, her other activities had not slowed down, her concentration was not impaired, her memory was not impaired, her thinking processes were all normal. There were no emotional symptoms: no crying, no look of sadness, no sense of agitation in the way she talked. Still, she had these maddening headaches.

There were two clues. She had trouble falling asleep at night, indicating an anxiety headache rather than one caused by depression. The other clue was in her responses to certain questions. The responses were too carefully controlled. But you had to look hard for cracks in the façade and closely for any change of pace in tone or amplitude.

"When," I asked, "did you first begin getting these headaches?"

"Just after we got married," she said. For just a moment, a vulnerability showed in her mouth and her voice. And then it passed.

As casually as possible—not emphasizing this exploration more than the conversation about other facts of her life—I explored her marriage.

She had met her husband, an up-and-coming young businessman, on one of her flights. They dated, fell in love, and decided to get married. It was as simple as the fable of flight that every young flight attendant cherishes. But somewhere, somehow, after that it all began coming apart. At least that's what the timing of her headache suggested. My questions were careful, yet it was not hard to see they had a central point. Did the marriage conflict in any way with the joy she'd gotten from her work? No. She'd left the airlines for a while after the wedding, but she'd returned recently and with no objection from her husband.

Was everything all right at work now? Yes.

Was there any in-law problem—were his parents beginning to get on her nerves? No, nothing like that.

How about the other way around did her parents have any kind of reservations about the man that she married? No, none that they'd ever expressed to her. They seemed to regard him as highly as she did.

How, in general, were she and her husband getting along? They were getting along fine—socially.

Interesting qualification, I thought.

So I began exploring the other aspects of the marriage. Were there any financial problems? No. Were there any conflicts of habit or temperament? No—nothing unusual. Were there any sexual problems? No. But again I thought I heard a vulnerability in her voice.

We wound up the first visit by exploring the potential of other stresses in the marriage.

It was clear that she wasn't ready to tell me what was bothering her, or else I just couldn't find the right questions. In any case, I prescribed a mild tranquilizer and suggested she come back and see me in two weeks.

She did, and I learned nothing except that the tranquilizers helped her get to sleep, if not to end the headaches.

We talked, not so exclusively about her marriage this time, but about some of the other factors that affected her daily life. It is the function of the physician, when dealing with chronic tension-type headache, to take a careful inventory not only of the patient's marital relationship but also her social and occupational relationships, her life stresses, her personality traits, and her habits in handling stressful situations. It requires a great deal of time to explore all of them, then to review again and again and reevaluate them each time to see what new clues might be uncovered.

And so, as she came to her appointments, I'd explore first how the pain was going and, if the situation demanded it, I'd change her prescription ever so slightly. Then we would sit and talk about any or all of the pertinent factors mentioned above. It often takes a long time for a doctor to win the confidence of his patient in such sensitive matters. And it was particularly difficult with this patient. For with all her apparent spontaneity, I got the feeling that in certain of these matters she had built her defenses high and deep. And I was not able to penetrate them.

Then one day she came in, distraught instead of cool. The pain in her head was intense and she walked somewhat stiffly, with her shoulders high, as if hunched against some anticipated blow. As I came into the examining room, she stood up and looked at me with a small defiant face. This was the moment, I knew, when I would get at the cause of the headache.

It came out slowly at first. It happened the night before. Not for the first time. Not, she feared, for the last. It was sex. *Of course*, it was sex. She and her husband had started in the sex act but, in all the months she'd been married, they'd never completely consummated their marriage. Her blue eyes swam out of focus and then came back, shocked and wide and full of tears which choked her. But the story came out piece by piece.

She and her husband would begin to make love. She would be intensely aroused. He would be intensely aroused. But then as they neared the climax, he would suddenly withdraw and go to the bathroom.

Time after time it had happened. All these months she'd feared that there was something wrong with her as a sexual partner. She wasn't able to attract or keep her husband close to her long enough to come to a climax. She had developed a constant anxiety about this, and the anxiety was manifested in an intense and recurring headache.

But the night before had been particularly traumatic. After her husband had left their bed, she gathered up the courage to burst in on him in the bathroom. There she found him stark naked, completing the sex act along while staring at a picture of a naked girl in a magazine.

The story came out in spasms, in rushes or words. I wondered if she had really cried since her wedding night. But now the torment was deepened.

84

She was ridding herself of a kind of poison, coughing it out. It took her a long time to tell her story. When finally it was all over, she settled into that preternatural calm that so often follows a violent outburst.

We talked quietly. I had discovered the cause of the headache, and there was no medicine and no chemistry that would cure it. But here were words, logic, reason, and the obvious. The problem, I told her, was not with her. It was with him. There was, as far as I could see, nothing wrong with her sexually. But *he* had a serious problem.

I urged that he—not she, as she'd feared—get psychiatric guidance. In fact, I volunteered to intercede for her, to talk to him, and try to persuade him to seek guidance. It was, of course, an extraordinary effort for a headache specialist, and was a futile one. He came to see me, and he did not receive the suggestion well. In fact, he seemed disturbed that his sexual aberration had been made known to a physician.

His bride turned out have a strong streak within her. She confronted him with his refusal and told him that she could not continue in the marriage unless and until he sought psychiatric help. He did nothing about it. And so one day I was asked to help in some of the religious details of her separation. She was a Roman Catholic, and she was going to get an annulment, not a divorce. I filed an affidavit with the Archdiocese attesting to the facts that had been revealed to me. She received the annulment after less than a year of marriage. And a year or so later she entered into a more regular and fulfilling marriage.

Her headaches? Well, they were rooted in an anxiety, which she kept locked within her for so many months. Once the key was turned, the emotions flowed out. Her headache ended after the deeply emotional scene in my office.

9

THE MYSTERIOUS MIGRAINE

It was a mystery without a clue, a riddle without an answer. The young woman had come to our office at the suggestion of her family physician. We gave her the basic in-office physical examination, which eliminated any organic problem, and we recorded her personal and case history.

Everything pointed to a migraine without aura. She reported a family history of migraine. The pain settled in the forehead (although it sometimes attacked both sides of the head, not just one, as is so often the case in migraine). The pain was pounding in nature and, although she had no aura, during the headache she was very sensitive to light and sound.

But the headache had no pattern. It did not always come at her menstrual period; sometimes she would go for months without a headache. It turned out that she'd been on and off birth control pills for several years (she was now 21). She'd been off them for eight months recently and had felt no headaches then. She was seized again by pain when she resumed taking them. But that had not made much of an impression on her.

Few women know that migraine can be triggered by a change in concentration of female hormones and that birth control pills increase this concentration. When a woman starts a birth control pill, there is a one-third chance headaches will worsen, but there is also a one-third chance the headaches will improve. In the remaining one-third of patients, the headache stays the same. So, if a patient who is taking a birth control pill is having an extremely difficult time managing her migraine, then we may recommend she stop taking the Pill. Conversely, if a woman who is not taking birth control begins to take birth control, she has a one-third chance that her headaches will improve. There is still, however, the chance they will worsen or stay the same.

The change in estrogen levels, specifically the fall in estrogen concentration that occurs just before a menstrual period begins, is thought to be a major trigger of migraine. Estrogen is thought to be one of the predominant reasons that migraine is so much more common among women than men. Oral contraceptives are distributed with placebo pills, which, when taken, precipitate a drop in estrogen concentration in the body (because they do not contain estrogen like the active drug pills do), which in turn allows the patient to have a menstrual period. In many cases, however, this drop in estrogen triggers migraine. In these cases we have a few options to consider. We can either ask the patient to skip the placebo days and continue with active drug, thus preventing the drop in estrogen and the trigger for migraine, or we can recommend a birth control pill such as Seasonique that allows for the drop in estrogen and a menstrual period only once every three months. By preventing the drop in estrogen and the resulting menstrual period, we can often also prevent a very real migraine trigger two out of every three months.

Because of the increased risk of stroke associated with estrogen-containing products such as oral contraceptives, it is recommended that if a patient with migraine with aura is prescribed a contraceptive that the lowest dose of estrogen possible, or even a progesterone-only product, is considered. This is due to the further increased risk of stroke that is seen in patients with migraine with aura. There are varying guidelines on this, from the International Headache Society's recommendation that women with migraine with aura should be allowed a low-dose estrogen contraceptive, to the World Health Organization (WHO) guidance that estrogen-containing contraceptives are contraindicated in women with migraine with aura.

Low-dose estrogen contraceptives are generally a better idea for migraine patients for another reason. Low-dose estrogen contraceptives have been shown to have a lower incidence of headache as well. In addition to low-dose estrogen, other contraceptive options for women with migraine with aura include progesterone-only contraceptive pills, a progesterone or copper intrauterine device (IUD), a progesterone implant, or a progesterone injection.

Not terribly long ago, for example, I examined a patient in her 30s who had just suddenly come down with a severe migraine. It seemed to attack her waking hours, and it was growing in intensity. I confirmed that it was migraine, but I couldn't determine why she had it or why it attacked her so suddenly and with such ferocity. But the basic function of the headache specialist is to quell the pain, even if he or she can't pinpoint the basic cause of the headache.

So, we prescribed the medications, we tried the special diet, and we didn't have to consider taking her off of the Pill because she'd never been on it. She was in her 30s, and she observed both a personal and religious discipline regarding sex.

But nothing we recommended or prescribed seemed to work. Her headaches continued as frequently and painfully as ever.

It was a baffling case because everything should have fallen into place and nothing did. It is the particular fortune of our office that we get only the tough cases; the easy ones are taken care of by nonspecialists. But that is no consolation when you're faced with an apparently insoluble mystery.

Then one day we were talking things over when I glanced at her personal as well as her medical history, and I noticed that she worked for a drug company.

"They're famous for their birth control pills," I commented casually.

"Yes," she said. "I know. I work in the section where we process the powder so that it can be made into a pill."

Voila! That was it!

As she worked and breathed, she inhaled some of those tiny air-suspended particles from which the birth control pills are made. In fact, she must have been inhaling enough of the chemical powder from working in that room all day to touch off a basic effect of the Pill—to increase the concentration of female hormones in her body. And that touched off the migraine headaches—

which she was prone to but had never quite suffered before. So, with her permission, I wrote to the company to see if she could be assigned to another department. She was reassigned, and her headaches ceased altogether shortly thereafter.

Beyond all this, the impact of the elements in the Pill exposes migraine patients to complications which might escalate into problems of dramatic proportions. There is an increased risk of stroke in migraine patients over the general population, and that risk is even higher in patients with migraine with aura.

The migraine type in which researchers first discovered patients had an increased risk of stroke was hemiplegic migraine. Medically, it can be said to occur when the patient experiences partial paralysis of one side of the body. It is often thought to be a stroke, but it is rarely so serious, or permanent, as that. It is more often a migraine complication masquerading as a stroke.

In fact, I first noticed hemiplegic migraine in an elderly patient who should have long been over her migraine attacks. She'd lived with migraine for 50 years and now she was 65-years old and nature had played a dirty trick on her: the migraines had increased in the previous two or three years but now they were attacking at the rate of two or three a week, a very high frequency.

Certainly there was an explanation for it. She had begun taking hormone replacement therapy when she passed through menopause some 20 years earlier, and she was still taking them. Migraine declines after menopause largely because there is a decrease in the secretion of female hormones in the body. (And it is the change in hormones—during menstruation, for example— that helps to trigger the migraine attack. Similarly, it is an increase in the concentration of female hormones as stimulated by the Pill that triggers a migraine attack in Pill takers who are susceptible to migraine.) But there was no natural decrease in female hormones in this patient after menopause because she was taking female hormone pills, and thus there was no decrease in or disappearance of her migraine.

She refused to give up the hormones because she feared a loss of femininity. Many patients, who are told to stop using birth control pills or hormones, will not follow their physician's advice, although we find that hormones can, in fact, sometimes be a culprit.

For 15 months, we managed to control her headaches, largely through use of triptans. But the day after Christmas one year, she phoned me in a state of near panic. Yes, she had migraine pain, but it was much more than that. She had developed a paralysis of her right arm and her right leg. She was convinced that she had suffered a stroke and that the headache might have been more than a migraine. It might have been a blood vessel breaking—the brain hemorrhage that is the cause of a stroke.

I had her admitted to the hospital as an emergency case. We ran through some neurological examinations and, sure enough, there was evidence of a "neurological deficiency." Her knee and arm reflexes on the right side were affected and there was a positive Babinski reading in her right foot. The big toe bent upward when the bare sole of her foot was stroked instead of bending downward.

We started treatment immediately, of course. I tried to encourage her by assuring her that she'd recover completely. She pretty much let me know that I had more confidence in her condition than she did. There was a reason for my confidence. I believed that she had not, in fact, suffered a stroke but a severe episode of hemiplegic migraine.

As it turned out, my diagnosis was correct. The patient recovered readily and swiftly from her paralysis and soon reached the point where there was no evidence that she'd ever had a stroke. She hadn't, of course. The migraine, being deeply involved with the blood vessels around the brain, had merely caused a complication that duplicated the appearance of a stroke. Through medication and by persuading her to give up her hormones, we managed to keep her at this point from getting so severe a migraine—or, for that matter, from suffering anything but a very mild and incipient migraine.

We recommended strongly to the 21-year-old woman who had started taking the Pill again that she give it up. In her case, the Pill clearly made her migraine worse. We also put her on the special diet, to avoid foods containing chemicals (tyramine and its near relative phenethylamine) that tend to trigger migraine in the migraine-prone (see p. 268). We prescribed zolmitriptan (Zomig), a triptan, which she could take to abort, or interrupt, the headaches once they got started. We knew pain, not an aura, was going to be her first signal that a migraine attack was coming. So in order to make the drug effective quickly, we prescribed the drug in a nasal spray form, which provides swifter action than from swallowing it.

She came back after a month, worse than ever, so we switched both strategy and tactics. Instead of trying to interrupt the headache after it started, we decided to try to prevent it from getting started. We put her on a daily intake of propranolol (Inderal). Then we gave her an injectable form of sumatriptan to see if we could quell the pain once it got started.

That worked all right, except that now she began getting her headaches regularly during her period. So we added an anti-inflammatory medication, naproxen, that she could take for three days before and during her period, and that worked well for two months. She visited me several times and seemed encouraged. Then right after the last visit the headaches increased in both severity and frequency. We were totally mystified. The headaches had proven stubborn from the start, but bit by bit we'd managed to get them under control. Now they were much worse than before she'd ever come to us.

The only thing we could do was switch medications and their dosages again. I prescribed the antidepressant amitriptyline (Elavil), which often diminishes migraine. I had done the original research work on Elavil in the late 1960s and early 1970s, and it is still the most frequently used drug to control chronic pain.

As it happened, she did very poorly on it. As the deadline approached, her headaches seemed to become more severe and intense. Naturally, locked in pain for so long, her sense of confidence in me and in the treatment began to erode, and still I had no answer to the mystery.

At this point the doctor must ask himself some very basic questions. Were we wrong in diagnosing a migraine headache? If so, what other kind of headache could it be? If we were wrong, what type of treatment is recommended? If we were right, was there some other kind of treatment that should be recommended? We took her off all medications for a short while. I looked at everything we'd done as objectively as possible. It just did not seem to me that we'd been wrong in our diagnosis. The evidence was strong that migraines were attacking her (though the frequency of some of her later attacks suggested they were overlaid with depression). So I started her again on a drug that she could take before and during her menstrual cycle, this time naratriptan. Then I discovered, by a casual question, the reason for it all. She was back on the Pill.

Moreover, she was back on it because of one of the nurses in our office, one new to our operation, told her to do it. "I wouldn't get off the Pill if I were you," she told the patient. We solved the whole problem with swift and simple action and fired the nurse. We got the patient to promise to give up the Pill. We took her off all drugs except for an antidepressant for temporary use. And we saw her headaches diminish and finally disappear.

This most plaguing and baffling of mysteries was solved by one of the simplest and most direct of actions: finding out if the patient is following the doctor's orders.

10

THE ONCE-A-MONTH HEADACHE

Grace Walters had missed some important, and even some not-so-important events during the past 17 years of her life because of debilitating headache pain. She could live with the missed work days, dinner parties, luncheons, bridge club meetings, and more, but what she couldn't forget, despite how trivial it seemed now, was having missed the junior prom when she was 16 years old because she was sick in bed with a headache. Why would this particular event remain so vividly etched in her memory? Obviously, the junior prom meant a lot to a bright, popular young teenager like Grace Walters. But perhaps the prom stayed in her memory because this was precisely the time when her headache problem began. Since that awful first headache when she was 16, each and every month—always during her menstrual period—Grace Walters had experienced a sickening migraine headache complete with nausea and vomiting that left her bedridden the last three days of her menstrual flow. (Age 16 was the start of her headache problem even though her period had started three years earlier.)

Now 33 years old, Grace Walters had come to believe that one week out of the month she would be sick as a result of her headaches. And as if that wasn't enough in itself, she also suffered terrible abdominal cramping the first two days of her period. In comparison to the headaches, though, her abdominal cramping wasn't all that bad—a heating pad and a little aspirin kept it from being much of a problem. The headaches were entirely another matter.

Unfortunately, Grace Walters' family had offered her little hope through these years of pain. Her mother, who had lived like this as well during her reproductive years, suffering similar one-sided headaches, merely told her daughter that this was the burden she had to accept with being a woman. Her husband, on the other hand, had basically come to accept the fact that this was her "time of the month" and his time to shuttle ice packs and pain pills to his bedridden wife, and help with the cooking. Like many migraine sufferers, she was also compulsive. After a large party she had given on a day she had a headache, she diligently washed her dishes on one side of the sink while vomiting into the other side of the sink. Over the years, her family doctor had given her a variety of medications to treat the pain, none of which proved to be very successful. Out of desperation, she finally sought more help and found our Headache Clinic.

The menstrual migraine Grace Walters suffered is one of the most common forms of migraine headache. Nearly 70 percent of all migraine victims are women and about 70 percent of these women experience their headaches immediately before, during, or after their menstrual flow. This is due to the change in estrogen concentration, notably the decrease in estrogen, that occurs during this time. It should also be noted that by the third month of pregnancy, most women become free of their migraine, except for a very small number who get their first attack with pregnancy. In addition, the estrogens contained in birth control pills or postmenopausal hormones can also be precipitating factors in a migraine attack. Remember that when a woman starts a birth control pill, there is a one-third chance headaches will worsen, but there is also a one-third chance the headaches will improve. In the remaining one-third of patients, the headache stays the same.

In Grace Walters' case, I tried to help with her migraine as well as her menstrual cramps. I prescribed a nonsteroidal anti-inflammatory medication, ibuprofen. This medication is a prostaglandin inhibitor. It was developed to help treat the type of menstrual cramps from which she suffered. These same types of chemicals, prostaglandins, seem to be involved in causing the headaches that are brought on by the hormonal changes responsible for the menstrual flow. Thus, this medication helps prevent the migraine attacks as well as the abdominal pain. In addition to ibuprofen, the three other nonsteroidal anti-inflammatory agents that have proven to be effective in treating menstrual migraine are flurbiprofen, naproxen sodium (Naprosyn), and Ponstel (mefenamic acid). These drugs were discovered and their use defined by a good friend of mine, Sir John Vane of the British Isles, and he received the Nobel Prize for Medicine for the discovery in 1982. Our family spent some very nice times with him and his wife in Venice, Chicago, and London. If the patients do not respond to the nonsteroidal anti-inflammatory agents, naratriptan or frovatriptan can be given twice daily during the menstrual period to prevent menstrual migraine.

Grace Walters started taking the ibuprofen three days before her next menstrual flow began and stayed with it until the end of her flow. Happily, she found that the menstrual cramps she usually experienced during the first two days of her menstruation had subsided. She awoke with trepidation on the third day of her flow since this was usually the day in which her headache emerged. The seemingly endless years in which she had suffered this monthly headache had understandably left her fearful of this day. It was, however, uneventful. She had taken her pills and was able to live a normal day and enjoy a nice dinner with her husband without the slightest trace of a headache. The next day wasn't quite so good, however, since she awoke with a mild headache. But after breakfast and even after lunch, the headache still remained mild and never required her to miss any of her activities.

This pattern continued over the following months and years, and now the headaches are truly a part of her past.

11

MAN'S MOST TERRIBLE PAIN

"It was early fall and I was driving home from my office in the city to the suburbs when about halfway home I began to get a headache of such magnitude that it became impossible to concentrate on driving. I pulled over to the side of the road and—still seated, even captured, behind the wheel—I began to writhe in pain. Holding my aching head, I hoped no one would stop because if I told them I had 'only' a headache they would think me insane for such carrying on."

In these words—simple, direct, free from hyperbole—Barry Chiant told of the onset of one of the most terrifying of headaches: the cluster headache. He was 34 years old when it first struck, a big, outgoing man, filled with the sense of his own being. He was big-boned, hard-muscled, a man of the outdoors with sun-squint eyes, a cheerful, seamed face, and powerful, clever hands. Yet he was reduced to helplessness by a cluster headache. This type of headache occurs 2, 3, or 4 times a day, sometimes even 6 to 10 times a day; thus, it comes in clusters. The pain comes on for 30 minutes or perhaps 1 to 2 hours, then it subsides only to return hard and maddening in a new headache a few minutes later. These clusters of pain do not go on month after month, year after year (except in a very few, very unfortunate individuals). Usually, the cluster headaches continue for a few weeks to a few months, say three to twelve weeks. Then they go away and the patient is pain-free for many months and he thinks the whole terrible episode is over. He's wrong. The headaches attack again a few months later, last for a time, then go away again. There is actually considerable pain-free time in the lives of cluster victims. Long or short periods of remission can occur within clusters. But when it happens, the pain so possesses and torments them that they hardly remember the time when there was no pain.[3]

---

[3] In the book *Headache Godfather*, we talk about a patient who sued me (Dr. Diamond) because he obtained a remission with an ambiguous treatment.

99

"After the pain subsided to nothing more than a dull, thud, I managed to continue driving home. Upon my arrival home, I was completely sapped and drained from experiencing this intense pain. I immediately went to bed. Unfortunately, lying down did not seem to help, and I began to experience another onset of pain."

The pain of a cluster headache is very intense indeed. It literally makes strong men weep. The hard specifics come from Dr. John Graham of the Faulkner Research Center in Boston, who reported that 32 percent of a group of cluster victims that he studied wept because of the pain; some 37 percent yelled out loud, 16 percent banged their heads on the wall, while another 14 percent fell to the floor and rolled and writhed in pain. It is this kind of pain that, we believe, led ancient man to have holes cut in his skull (trepanning) to let the pain—the evil spirits—out. Modern man seeks to escape the pain in less savage ways: one cluster victim will stick his head in an oven, another in a refrigerator, still another in a bucket of ice. But there is always the danger that the pain will drive its victims to suicidal extremes. "My wife took the shotgun out of our house," one cluster victim told me, "because she was afraid I might use it."

"After seeing what intense pain I was in," continued Barry Chiant, "my wife called an MD, a neighbor and a close friend of ours. He arrived within minutes and examined me and asked numerous questions. I described the location of the pain. It was in only one quarter of my head, from the middle of my skull forward to my mouth, and only on the right side. I described the tenseness of the muscles of my neck, the ringing of my right ear, and the clogged nasal passage."

The doctor, an allergist, gave him a shot to quiet him down. He diagnosed the problem, correctly, as a cluster headache. But he suggested that Barry Chiant consult a neurologist to make sure the pain was a cluster headache and not something else. "That 'else' became an obsession with me since one of my wife's best friends was then in the hospital suffering from a terminal brain tumor," he said.

At the Diamond Headache Clinic, cluster headache patients who phone for help get in as soon as possible. Normally, we're booked weeks in advance, but when the cluster victim phones, we upset the schedule and try to book him or her for immediate examination because the pain is so severe. Understandably, many doctors who don't specialize in treatment of the headache, or who don't appreciate the severity of cluster headaches, work cluster victims in through their regular scheduling system. In Barry Chiant's case, this meant waiting for 10 days. "The 10 days until I could get the appointment with the neurologist were living hell," he said. "The headaches kept recurring and now were as frequent as three a day." This meant that he'd have to take time off from work. Nobody can work with intense pain coming this frequently. He had his own business, a small communications agency dealing mostly in publications and advertising in the industrial field. So he could take time off when he needed it but only as long as the pressure of his work was not greater than the pain in his head. In the case of a cluster headache, the pressure of work would never overtake the pain in his head.

The neurologist gave him a full examination consisting of X-rays, brain scans, and so forth, and with them the assurance that he had no brain tumor. To control the headaches, the neurologist prescribed sumatriptan. The idea was that the headaches would get a start on him but perhaps, through the medication, he would be able to overcome them.

When the attacks went away altogether, Barry Chiant felt that he'd been successfully treated. He didn't know until five months later that they go away only for a time and then come back more fiercely than ever.

"My headaches returned in February," he said. He went back to the neurologist, who, quite logically, prescribed the same regimen as before. This time it didn't work quite as well; the neurologist changed the prescription somewhat. But when the headaches still seemed to dominate his patient's life, he suggested that perhaps Barry Chiant had been working too hard, was under too much stress, and should get away from it all for a while. As a matter of fact,

Barry Chiant was well past the busy season, but he was susceptible to the suggestion.

"About this time, a friend invited me to come to Florida," he said. "We'd sail over to the Bahamas and fish. Great! I thought. Here is my vacation. Sun, sea, and sand—what better way to get rid of the winter doldrums!" And, he hoped, everything else that bothered him. There was one very real problem: the vacation would not necessarily help him overcome his headaches.

To be sure, a great many people believe that cluster headaches are tied to the stress of business. "I didn't stop to think that in my busiest season, when I was under very considerable pressure, I didn't seem to get the headaches at all," said Barry Chiant. Indeed, it now appears that cluster headaches are perhaps the only headache that is not somehow connected to the emotions. Thus the emotional response to stress is not a trigger to cluster headache.

Barry Chiant found out about this the hard way. "Armed with my pills—just in case—I flew to Florida," he said. "We went on board the yacht." They weighed anchor. They cruised the blue-green waters of the Bahamas— lime green near the island shoals, turquoise in the depths, and he began getting severe headaches once again. "What is this?" he thought. "Here I am completely relaxed, doing what I love most, and I'm getting these insufferable headaches." The experience so shook him that, when he got home, he set off on a search for a cure for the headache—not just an occasional quelling of the pain.

"First, I went to my ophthalmologist for a checkup to see if my glasses needed changing," he said. "They did and when I asked her if this could be the cause of the headaches, she said she doubted it. She said I would outgrow them." To a man in his middle 30s, the only response was a sardonic one: "When?"

Next he went to the dentist. His teeth were okay. The dentist said there was no possible link to the headaches.

"Once more I called my allergist friend," he went on. "He seemed to know as much and perhaps more about these headaches, since he'd called the shot right off the bat. I asked him if these headaches could be triggered by an allergic reaction. He said, 'Maybe.'" Barry Chiant had already been looking into the possibility, and so he was keeping a record of everything he ate and, at the same time, keeping a record of when and where the headaches struck. "By trying to compare the two lists, I hoped to find if there was a cause in the food and an effect in the headache," he said. He suspected it was the Italian food that he loved to eat—with beer or wine, of course. He thought he saw a link between the timing of the food and pain. So he arranged to take a battery of allergy tests under the doctor's supervision, but there wasn't one thing I was allergic to!" I do find that smoking and any alcoholic beverages will provoke cluster headaches.

There was almost a note of despair in this. For the pain of cluster is so great that the search for a cure assumes the dimension of that for the Holy Grail. I had one patient who had his molars extracted, thinking that would stop the pain of cluster. I even had one who went through head surgery three times to stop the pain. These methods all failed. The latter is on the faculty of a business school in one of the nation's major universities. Some 35 or more years ago, when he was in his early 30s, he first suffered a cluster headache. It was first identified in 1867 as a headache different from migraine and from other headaches, but the most valuable research in the field has been done since 1936. By and large, that research was led by Dr. Bayard T. Horton of the Mayo Clinic. For that reason, the headache has been called Horton's syndrome. (It's also known by a number of other names such as migrainous neuralgia and, because it's been associated with the histamine level in the blood, as histamine cephalalgia.) It is thought to be a vascular headache; the pain is caused by a dilation, or swelling, of the blood vessels in the affected area.

There is a genetic predisposition to cluster headache. First-degree relatives are 5 to 18 times more likely to have cluster headache than the general population. Episodic cluster headache cycles range from two weeks to three months at a time, usually with one to several attacks per day or every other day. Chronic cluster headache is diagnosed when a patient continues to have cluster

103

headaches for more than one year, with less than a one-month period without attacks.

But at the time the professor, my patient, began suffering cluster headaches, the treatment tended to be either nonexistent or radical, and his was radical. In 1950, a doctor decided that the best way to end the pain was through surgery: he recommended the ligation of the left temporal arteries. Remember our discussion of the pain in the temporal arteries (see Chapter 5: "The Painful Hat")? Well, this doctor decided that by tying off, ligating, the left temporal arteries so that blood could not flow through them, he'd end the pain of the headache. He was wrong, however, the cluster headache continued; it simply switched over to the right side.

Next, the professor went to another doctor, who recommended another operation to cut certain nerves in the neck. It's called a cervical sympathectomy—a cutting of the sympathetic nerve chain in the neck, which controls certain blood vessels. That didn't work either.

In fact, the cluster pains let up only mildly from time to time; he is one of those unfortunate victims who never got complete relief from the attack. It was simply a case of a patient having an ailment which the doctors didn't completely understand, and so they tried to treat it in an innovative way. Not until we got him on a hard-hitting discipline of several drugs to prevent headaches and to abort them when they started did he get any relief, and even that was not complete. He still had the headaches, but he learned how to keep them under control.

Back to the case of Barry Chiant. He turned his search inward. Frustrated in his search of a medical cure, he began to look at his life to see if there was a clue to the sudden onslaught.

"How could I suddenly get these headaches and then go for months without a sign of them?" he asked. "I examined my life and found it pretty much in order. I was somewhat successful in business, did not worry too much, knew how to play, to enjoy myself, and in general led a busy, active, happy life. I participated in community affairs, had many fine friends, enjoyed many hobbies, and led a happy home life. I am the picture of a man who loves life and tries to live every moment of it. Then why the headaches? Certainly, they weren't a relief valve telling me to slow down. They occurred even when I was slowing down or was on vacation."

The man who came to us that day had much of the typical look of the cluster victim. For these headaches very often strike men whom we normally think of as having rugged, athletic, even virile good looks. They are strong-chinned, square-jawed men, quite often with a dimple in the chin, a la Cary Grant, and furrows in the forehead. Their lower lip is often well chiseled. They tend to have thick skin on their face. Often it is rough, or pitted, like the skin of an orange. You may notice a gathering, or conglomeration, of what seem to be all too apparent little veins on the nose and elsewhere on the face. The interesting and baffling thing is that even women who suffer from cluster headache have, in general, certain of these same facial conditions. At the time when this book was first written heavy smokers were quite prevalent, especially in cluster headache patients, and some of these facial changes may have been due to the heavy smoking. Although rates of smoking have decreased in the general population since this book was first published, smoking—or a history of smoking—continue to be quite common among cluster headache patients.

Barry Chiant was a painfully authentic version of the typical cluster victim. The cluster victim typically finds one of his eyes watering and one of his nostrils clogged up on the side where the pain comes. The pain, as we've seen, develops on only one side of the head—the medical term is unilateral. Indeed, it is often described as an intense, boring pain focused behind one eye or the other. (In Barry Chiant's case, it was the right eye.) Many patients get a slight warning of the onset of the headache; they have a faint discomfort or a slight burning sensation on the side where the pain comes.

The fact that Barry Chiant suffered his first attack while driving is, perhaps, slightly unusual. Now we know that many of these attacks take place during normal daytime activities simply because there are so many attacks in the course of a 24-hour period. But a great many patients seem to remember the initial attack, certainly the first of the day, as coming during the night and awakening them from a sound sleep. The pain is so sudden and intense that the calm of night and of sleep is turned into a blazing inferno of pain. The victim gets up and starts walking the floor—sometimes crying, sometimes screaming, and, as we have seen, sometimes writhing and rolling on the floor.

Because of the nighttime (and sleep time) onslaught, it is often hard to prevent that first attack of the day with an oral medication. With the pain of a cluster headache, probably more than with any other pain known to man, it is imperative to get relief as soon as possible. That is why in most cases medication is delivered either by injection or nasal spray. Sumatriptan can be administered subcutaneously and intranasal, while zolmitriptan is available in an intranasal formulation. These options provide much quicker relief for cluster headache than any of the oral triptans.

The hallmark treatment of cluster headache, however, is oxygen. High-flow oxygen, delivered via a face mask (and not by nasal cannula, which is what most people envision when they think of oxygen therapy). Generally within 15 minutes, the high-flow oxygen will abate the cluster attack. In some cases, both a triptan as well as oxygen is needed. Most cluster patients will have oxygen tanks in their homes during a cluster cycle so that they are able to treat their headaches when they occur.

The use of oxygen was first described by Horton and a friend of mine, Dr. Walter Alvarez at the Mayo Clinic in the mid-1960s. The neurological community active in headache at that time never really accepted its value. A headache practitioner, Lee Kudrow, father of actress Lisa Kudrow, in his publications on cluster revived its usefulness and helped promote its acceptance in the 1980s. Its use at the Diamond Headache Clinic also helped to promote its acceptance as a first-line treatment for cluster headache.

There are, of course, additional treatments for cluster headache. Sometimes, the use of lidocaine or cocaine in the form of nose drops will help intractable cases. There are also external devices that have been developed to stimulate the vagus nerve, and the results from clinical trials suggest these will provide additional options for cluster headache patients.

If the pain is quite severe, I'll use the corticosteroids on some patients, particularly prednisone and dexamethasone (Decadron). Another oral medication option is indomethacin, which is a nonsteroidal anti-inflammatory drug (NSAID). Indomethacin has been shown to be effective at lessening the duration and severity of a cluster cycle in some patients. This particular medication has shown effectiveness in some of the rarer headache conditions that we encounter in headache medicine. Years ago, indomethacin was widely used to treat arthritis, but its tendency to cause stomach ulcers and kidney impairment have lessened its use in primary care. Still, it is a very effective medication in some conditions.

In addition, I prescribe methysergide maleate (Sansert) in fairly large doses, even as high as 12 to 16 milligrams a day. Unfortunately, we can no longer use this therapy in the United States. The manufacturer has stopped making it reportedly because of manufacturing difficulties. I personally believe that it was removed because of the irritant of trial lawyers in a product whose financial returns weren't sufficient to provide for their aggravation.

It is true that regular use of Sansert can cause, as a side effect, certain kidney and heart problems, and it cannot be used during pregnancy. Once the run of the clusters is over, whether in weeks or months, the use of Sansert must be discontinued. Often, I'll ask the patient to undergo another physical examination before resuming its use, in the expectation that the cluster will return in another few months. For the patient must be given a vacation from Sansert every four to six months and must be watched carefully to make sure he or she does not fall prey to the side effects. I tried all of these remedies, except oxygen inhalation and the lidocaine nose drips on Barry Chiant. It was slow and painful for him,

107

but we did manage to get his headaches under control, though not to end them. Nevertheless, he was not defeated by the slow progress. "I was able to meet other headache sufferers—it was an enlightening, even rewarding, experience to know that others have this problem, too," he said. "Best of all, I was given hope: hope that my suffering would be lessened, hope that tomorrow would be better, hope in the chance to try new methods and new drugs and know that they'll be changed immediately if they don't do the job."

But he wanted to find a more complete freedom, a method of living his life without even the fear of pain. For he could not know, when he went fishing or hunting or even on a business trip across the country if the pain would strike him suddenly again, as it had in Florida and the Bahamas. The only defense he had against it was the drugs, which he'd have to carry with him whenever he left home. Thus it was natural that he wanted to find another way to defend himself against a sudden onslaught of the pain. He did not want to interrupt his pleasure in play or his purpose in work.

The method we decided to use is called histamine desensitization. There is, today, considerable debate as to what part histamine plays in the pain of cluster. Certainly antihistamines, which we find in cold compounds, do nothing to ease the pain of cluster headache. But in the years after 1936, when insight into this problem was growing, the role of histamine was regarded paramount. One thing is indisputable: the level of histamine deposited in the blood and urine during a cluster is far higher than normal. This is confirmed simply by a study of the blood and urine of patients during cluster attack. And histamine might also be us the cause of the stuffed-up nostril and tearing eyes that the cluster victim usually suffers during an attack.

Actually, histamine is a chemical (an amine) found in virtually all tissue. It is produced by the action of decaying bacteria, which are always present in the body. It was discovered in ergot. It is a substance that the body produces to fight injury or infection or some other malfunction. Its action is, by and large, thought to be beneficial. But it becomes apparent to us only as a rogue

108

in the bodily processes. It's what causes the plaguing nose problems of a head cold or the runny nose of hay fever and other allergies. And it may be implicated—note I say "may" because of the worldwide debate now going on—in the pain of cluster.

There are some experts in the field of headache treatment who have not only accepted the theory of histaminic implications in cluster, but who rely on treatment based on that supposition. We often have relatively large numbers of cluster patients going through a process of histaminic desensitization. This is simply a process of gradually getting the body used to histamine, so that it doesn't flare up in the pain of cluster when a large amount of histamine suddenly appears.

The histamine therapy was originally used by Dr. Horton at Mayo Clinic successfully. Neurologists never really tested this therapy and never promoted its use. Some of Horton's fellows at Mayo Clinic used it with phenomenal success but it was a dying therapy. Dr. Robert Ryan, Sr. of St. Louis was one of Horton's students and a longtime friend. He asked me to come to St. Louis to see the therapeutic value of this therapy. I visited him, and incorporated it into my own fight to help cluster patients.

This was the process that I chose to use with Barry Chiant in his search for a more enduring defense against cluster. It was not an easy process for a busy businessman, for it demanded that he be admitted to our inpatient headache unit for a period of 10 to 12 days for intravenous therapy.

In the hospital headache unit, the patient has a IV bag of fluid hung next to his bed. This fluid is fed, drop by drop, into a vein in his arm—an intravenous feeding. The fluid, of course, contains the histamine in carefully measured amounts. The time that it takes for the histamine to run into the bloodstream is gradually increased from around four hours the first day until the 12th day when the entire dose of histamine can be received in perhaps 1 to 1½ hours.

"Needless to say," said Barry Chiant, "I was reluctant to spend the time on one process. And the thought of being stuck in the arm and being plugged into a bottle seemed like a helluva poor way to spend the day. But the alternative..."

Nevertheless, he did it and he grew to like it. "The nurses almost made it seem like fun. And the others in our 'club' shared stories of their problems and of the dead-end streets they followed until they came to the Diamond Headache Clinic. By sharing our good times and bad, we helped each other in many small ways.

"The histamine program worked for me in that it shortened the length of the cycle and reduced the intensity of the attacks. It also seemed to make the medication work better. Most of all it had a long-term impact. It was 14 months until my next attack.

"This time it took a little longer for the series to have an effect, and I was getting quite depressed," he said. But that is when the doctor must offer support that is more than medical; he must offer reassurance and share with his patient a determination that the pain can be overcome and the patient can go back to a normal life. Again, the desensitization process took effect and the cycle of pain ended. This time he went 15 months without another attack of cluster. Up to the time of this writing, he hasn't had a recurrence. "This year," he said, "I won't need these intravenous feedings because I'm managing well on a regimen of diet, sleep, some medication, and self-evaluation."

Most of all, he's emerged from these experiences with a new maturity and deeper understanding of the problems of human suffering.

"I know that perhaps I will have these cluster headaches all my life," he said. "I have resigned myself to the fact that it could really be worse. Like the diabetic, the problem can't be cured but it can be managed. My doctor has given me hope. The attacks are less frequent, less severe, less debilitating. I know more about the problem and can help myself overcome it sooner. I know that headaches will only last so long and then I'll feel fine again.

"I suppose it makes me more conscious of how great it feels just to be well every day—and not to have a headache."

12

THE TYPICAL ATYPICAL HEADACHE

"It's like getting hit by a bolt of lightning right through my head." That is how Diane Frost described the intense, nearly unbearable pain she had been forced to live with for the past six months. "There isn't any warning, just sharp, jabbing pain that can last for days at a time." Even more distressing and confusing was the fact that this excruciating pain in her head came not once or twice a day but 10 times or sometimes even 15 or 20 times a day. Her attempts at relieving the pain were almost entirely futile because it lasted such a short time—in most cases, just a few moments. By the time she could take some aspirin, the pain would be gone until the next jabbing session.

Diane Frost couldn't understand what was happening to her. Everything had been going so well: The job at the investment company was exciting and a great deal of fun, and she had been planning some new decorating ideas for her trendy new condominium. Perhaps out of frustration, she started keeping a full bottle of aspirin in her desk drawer at work and she would grab a few each time the pain hit. For the next couple of weeks she thought she had this problem licked since the pains didn't seem quite so bad and were less frequent. Unfortunately, her stomach was beginning to feel the effects of all the aspirin. She started to get a gnawing pain in the pit of her stomach when she would take the pills. It was at this time she decided to seek real help. She was tired of this bitter cycle of pain, pills, and new pains.

That week, a friend at work mentioned a recent newspaper article about headache and one of the doctors quoted in that article practiced in Chicago. Diane Frost called our clinic immediately to see if we could help her. We made arrangements to see her on the following Saturday since she indicated that she really hated to miss time from work.

113

During her first visit, Diane Frost made it clear that she wasn't the hysterical type, and that she didn't want to fuss with "a bunch of pills" for her headaches. She preferred a more natural route, especially in light of the problem she had developed with the aspirin. After taking a careful history, which included finding out everything I could about her pain, I discovered that many of these attacks would come on if she looked to her right and up a little bit. This was an important clue in my search for what was causing her pain.

Diane Frost's description of her pain—numerous short, jabbing, or ice pick-like pains in various locations throughout her head—was clearly a symptom of a syndrome known as cluster headache variant. Although this syndrome is not really new, it was unrecognized for a number of years. I published a journal article on it and revived interest in it although there was little acknowledgment from the neurological community. Cluster headache variant is a combination of three separate types of headaches. The first type is atypical cluster headache. These headaches are chronic and, like cluster headaches, occur several times a day. They are atypical in that they do not always occur over the eye, they may last all day long, and they shift from one location to another. The second type of headache involves the multiple, short, jabbing pains Diane Frost experienced. The third type of headache that these patients can experience is a background vascular headache, typified by a chronic or continuous one-sided headache of variable severity. This headache is vascular due to its throbbing nature—it is very intense. Cluster headache variant patients who exhibit two or three of these types of pain, have been responsive to a nonsteroidal, anti-inflammatory agent known as indomethacin (Indocin). I worked with indomethacin in the late 1960s and early 1970s before it was ever marketed. It was one of the first nonsteroidal anti-inflammatory agents (NSAIDs) and we examined its use in patients with osteoarthritis. Some of my other research with this drug found it effective for coital headache in the male and for both men and women who have exertional headache.

However, any individual who has cluster headache variant should always have a very thorough workup, including an MRI scan to make sure there is no organic cause for the pain.

I explained to Diane Frost the need to check her over completely to ensure that there was nothing seriously wrong. This included a complete examination of her nervous system as well as her neck. It was during this part of the exam that I triggered an attack by having her turn her head and neck to the right and up. With a sharp wince, she clenched her teeth and said, "Here it comes again." The pains subsided quickly, just it had during the previous attacks.

I recommended that she have an MRI to verify that there wasn't some underlying disease of the neck or skull at work here. I then explained to her that she was probably suffering from a form of vascular headache called cluster headache variant. Like cluster, it occurred multiple times a day, but unlike the typical cluster headache. I also had to explain that despite her aversion to taking a lot of pills, there wasn't a "natural way" to treat these headaches, and that it would require some medication. In any case, I realized that I would need to be very conservative in whatever medication I prescribed, so I asked her to take Indocin. Normally, I would have asked her to take a capsule of Indocin three or four times a day, but being aware of her reluctance to take a lot of medication, I gave her a form of the drug called Indocin SR (which stands for "sustained release"). This enabled her to take a single capsule or two per day and achieve the same beneficial results. I warned her, however, that the Indocin could cause her some stomach problems just as the aspirin had done, but that she could avert these problems by taking the medication with breakfast each day. I left her with a final piece of advice: to call me anytime if she had any problem with the medication or the headaches. Assured that I was willing to work with her, Diane Frost accepted the prescription.

After taking the Indocin over the next 48 hours, Her jabbing pains began to subside, and by the third day she was no longer getting them at all. She continued the prescription for another week to guarantee that the headaches were gone. However, she chose to test the medication's effectiveness, wondering if this all had been some sort of passing fad, and she stopped taking the Indocin. Within a day after stopping the medication, the pain returned. After another two days of headache pain, Diane Frost resumed taking the Indocin and again the pain stopped, but in this instance, it subsided the same day she started taking the capsules. This time she stayed with the prescription. During her next appointment at the Clinic, she told me about her experience with the medication and the headaches. I assured her this was rather typical for atypical cluster headaches.

13

THE MISTAKEN NEUROTIC

The tragedy is in the needless waste. Men and women live their entire lives in pain and find them wasted as they enter the twilight years. Somebody, somewhere, might have found the way to end that pain. Instead, the first doctor made a mistaken first judgment—that migraine was "all in the head," for example—and doomed the patient to a life of pain.

I'm thinking in particular of a woman, now in her 60s, who came to me after having endured headache pain for almost a half-century. "As far back as I can remember," she said, "I had such terrible sick headaches!" For most of those years the medical profession was not aware just what was involved in headache pain, so it tended to dispose of her rather than treat her. And it disposed of her by classifying her as neurotic, and as being emotionally unstable, because she had a pain in her head that could not be explained at that time.

Stacia Stephan was, by the time I first met her, a colorless, short, overweight woman with glasses and a somewhat pinched nose, as if she'd smelled something distasteful. She had begun getting migraine headaches as a little girl, and they continued all through her teens. They got worse after she was married at the age of 21. Both her parents and her husband set out with her on a round of doctors, none of whom could do much to overcome the headaches.

"They kept telling me it was just nerves, or I just *thought* I had headaches," she said. "To them, it was all mental." But the reality of pain was affecting her mental state. "I often thought I was going out of my mind, they hurt so." The familiar pattern of migraine pain dissolved into the daily pattern of an inescapable pain. "Night after night, I would wake up with terrible pain at 4 or 5 o'clock in the morning," she said.

She became aware of the Headache Clinic, made an appointment, and arranged to have her latest doctor send her medical records, just on the chance there was a hint of organic difficulty in her pain, which there wasn't.

She had actually been suffering two different kinds of headaches for many years. One was the original migraine. But as this continued to attack her year after year, she developed chronic daily headache, largely due to depression. You can appreciate how and why she might develop depression when faced with the expectation of pain. And the expectation, in encouraging depression, itself became pain.

Since her treatment from other doctors had not been effective with the tricyclic antidepressants such as amitriptyline (Elavil), I prescribed the monoamine oxidase inhibitor (MAOI), phenelzine sulfate (Nardil). As discussed earlier, we only use it in very compliant patients and only if other treatments have failed. Many doctors have a fear of using it due to either lack of experience or not appreciating how it can help in refractory depression. It is a mood elevator that can help break the grip of depression. It also has the capability of blocking the migraine attack. The medication appeared to work. Her headaches lessened, then disappeared. It was the depression headache that succumbed first. The migraine lost its hold, perhaps because she'd already passed through menopause.

In any case, she had gone three years without a severe headache that last time I talked with her. But she was now over 60 years old. She'd been married for almost 40 years. Her life, which might have been elevated by a sense of personal fulfillment, instead had been needlessly, tragically, and wastefully racked by pain.

118

14

THE NEAR-MADDENED MISSIONARY

One would like to think that there is justice in the workings of nature. If so, it isn't apparent in the workings of headache pain. For migraine, in particular, strikes the strivers and doers in society, and sometimes it strikes those who are trying to make great contributions. I was reminded of this not long ago when I looked over the medical record of one of my patients, Abigail Dalton. She was a missionary in Africa, and during her years of missionary work her toil was made even more difficult by remorseless attacks of migraine.

The headaches struck first when she was a teenager and continued all through her adult years. She married and raised three children. She and her husband entered church work and then missionary work. In their 40s and 50s, they labored in mission work in Africa. They led active lives, seeking to understand the African culture of their mission and the Western culture of their church. But it was a labor that was continually marred by pain—the migraine that she suffered. Even the simplest of acts was interrupted by it. She can recall riding with her husband in the family car the 1,050 miles from her post in Zimbabwe to Durban, South Africa—stretched out on the back seat, trying to mute the pain of her migraine.

Eventually, both she and the mission wondered if she could continue her work. The pain seemed almost maddening at times. The focus of missionary is, in its ideal, the giving of the human spirit. But pain draws one inward, away from people and away from giving. It became a question of whether the pain or the giving person who bore it would win.

The pain won. The woman decided to give up her work in Africa and come back home. Her husband joined her in the decision. Thus, we may see the injustice of pain—it took two people from their work, although only one person was stricken with pain.

The couple settled near Chicago, and one day, directed by mission headquarters, she sought out our Headache Clinic.

She was 54 years old when I first saw her. She had a number of small problems—with her eyes, her thyroid, fibrous (nonmalignant) cysts in a breast, and a family inclination toward diabetes (she was a borderline case). But her main problem was with headache pain.

She had migraine headaches, of course. And they had persisted well beyond menopause. One reason may have been that for several years she took hormone replacement therapy and they tended to stimulate the susceptibility to migraine. I prescribed propranolol (a beta blocker) to control the headaches. The medicine barely attacked the problem. A week later she came back, still bothered by pain. The reason was that she'd transformed to chronic migraine— brought about by a mixture of both depression and anxiety. This was understandable; it was a reaction to an expectation of pain. The psychogenic nature of the headache was exhibited not only in pain but in sleep. She was having trouble falling asleep and then staying asleep. The migraine medicine had not touched the daily headache, so after one or two more tries, I added an antidepressant to the prescription, amitriptyline (Elavil), and it seemed to do the job. I did my original work with amitriptyline (Elavil) in the late 1960s. It is a generic drug used by most headache physicians and neurologists to treat chronic migraine. This contribution to headache therapy is one of which I'm most proud. Many times the combination of two different drugs carefully adjusted can do the job in refractory patients. Her headache pattern began breaking up, and after her third visit she reported significant reduction in the frequency and pain of her headaches. The gratifying thing is that she used the reprieve to go right back into missionary work. Two months after her first visit to my office, she and her husband were on their way to Africa. She tested herself with an exceedingly busy round of activities in the United States, then with a 20-hour flight back to Africa. She was free of pain all this time—but she was stricken with a tormenting headache nine days after she arrived back in Zimbabwe. It came on

120

each morning for four straight days. But she moved up her time of consumption of the medicine and this seemed to work well. Perhaps it was in response to jet lag; by moving up the time of consumption in Africa, she was approaching more closely the time she consumed the medicine when in the United States.

Later she and her husband drove the 1,050 miles to Durban, and she made it without one attack of headache. But several days later she was stricken again and went to bed with a headache. We corresponded occasionally via e-mail, and I particularly enjoyed hearing about her adventures in Africa. Through the e-mails, however, I noticed that a certain pattern was emerging. She seemed to be getting the headaches after the strain of a long trip. This suggested that perhaps she was overloading her life—as migraine patients do—and that maybe she'd control the headache better if she did not try to fit too much in to her life at one time. We cannot, as I've already said, always end headache pain forever, but we can help the victim to control it—if she can control her own life and instincts.

She did just that, and she continued taking her medicine. Bit by bit, her headaches dwindled to a level at which they were first tolerable and then barely noticeable. For me it was a personal as well as professional satisfaction. For in returning this woman to her mission in Africa and helping her to work effectively there, we were doing a good turn for one who was constantly giving of herself.

15

THE WOMAN LIKE ALL OF US

When I came into the examination room, Anne Darby got up and gave me a kiss on the cheek. It took me aback. She was attractive, with tossed blonde hair, a laughing mouth, and seemingly endless energy and charm. She was also something other than what she seemed.

She came down from a medium-sized town in Indiana. She said she'd had headaches ever since she could remember. From the time before she first went to school she could "remember having what I thought were very bad head pains and crying for long times in a day. My parents explained them away, saying that child could not have headaches of such intensity." Now we know that children can have very severe migraine attacks, even at an age when they cannot really talk about or explain them. Anne Darby said, "Nothing was done for them at that time."

It was not apparent on that first visit, but those headaches had led her into a series of abysmal experiences. Yet there was no hint of any of that in the perky, pleasant manner with which she greeted me.

"I deliberately put on my most cheerful attitude," she told me later. "I didn't want you to think I was a neurotic or a hypochondriac. After years of pain, you begin to wonder if every doctor you see thinks you are neurotic. I am sure I'm not. I hate being ill. It interferes with my life as I want to live it."

It wasn't hard to see that she'd begun by having migraine. She still revealed the distinctive traits of the migraine personality. ("I must have some sort of project, if not two, in the fire. People who doodle irritate me, and wasting time when one could be productive infuriates me.") Over the years, she'd also transformed to chronic migraine, which was as least partly a result of long-term depression. Anne Darby was like most of us in her goals, hurts, fears, and apprehensions, but the way all these came together, with pain as their punctuation point, warped her life. She underwent experiences which can only be described as macabre. And yet they might have happened to anyone, given headache pain as a constant companion.

"The headache became a regular happening with my menstrual cycle, starting at age 11," she said. "There was no vomiting, but there was some nausea with a tendency to black out, as if I had risen from a 'down' position too quickly. Intense excitement or anger would bring on the blackouts or dizziness, and the headache would last a full day."

Two events tended to make them worse. They were ignored instead of treated. Anne Darby's mother was ill with cancer for several years, and up to her death, the whole focus of family life was around her mother and her mother's illness. So, in this perspective, it was understandable that the headache problem of a young girl might get lost in the enormous concerns for her mother.

When her mother died, Anne Darby's headaches became worse. At the same time, she did not have the understanding help of an older woman as she entered puberty. "I was a very shy, inward girl," she said. "Much of this was due to my physical appearance." She was a tall, thin, awkward girl. "My complexion was ever so pale—the pretty, blue-eyed blonde, I was not. Blonde, yes, but so were my eyelashes, which made for a startlingly blank face. When people say children can be cruel, it is true. But I do believe that the effects of adult comments about my appearance were the more jarring and long lasting." Time, and her father's remarriage, helped her adjust to these problems.

"As the ugly duckling became the swan, God took pity and gave me a sweet face that makeup could do wonders for. A stepmother, who took great pride in clothing my sister and myself in a most fashionable manner, also helped," she said. There were still, of course, social problems to be conquered.

"I had no friends, but there was a drive to be successful and popular. I took a close look at the personalities of the more popular girls and molded their better traits into my habits. It was a constant struggle not to slip back into my own shy personality, which had also been made more insecure with the added feeling of being unloved and physically ugly. To change all of these things did not seem to be too hard on the surface. I covered all with a laugh and a smile. I became known as a smiling, happy, outgoing person. Inside, of course, none of the fears had vanished, but I accomplished what I set out to do for myself and that was all that mattered. There was another fear on my list of insecurities now—the fear of anyone finding out my true self, whatever that was or is." She chose the familiar route of security so often blazed by the teenage girl.

"By 18 I was married. Success was still my goal, but with it was also a true belief in subservience and obedience as a wife. This added much stress to my marriage, for to be obedient (in the demands of her first marriage) I would have to give up what I thought success should be and I would have to change my moral principles."

In an attempt to make her marriage better, she became pregnant at 19. The migraine, unexpectedly, did not disappear during pregnancy; usually it is gone by the end of the second month of pregnancy. "During the pregnancy, my headaches became very frequent," she said. "I lived on pain-relieving drugs. In the latter part of the eighth month, I gained 20 pounds in three days. Then I had what was diagnosed as three grand mal seizures [of epilepsy] in a 12-hour period and went into a coma. The baby was delivered by cesarean section."

She came out of her coma after four days. She awakened to distressing news. "I was told by two specialists in neurology I had epilepsy." The shock was traumatic, the fear was even greater. "My visions of an epileptic were not too pleasant," she said.

The headaches became frequent now, only they were more violent, lasting up to three or four days with vomiting included. She said, "Between the seizures and the migraines, it was hard to keep smiling. Only once was I hospitalized with a migraine. The rest of the times I would go to the emergency room at the hospital and would be given a shot that would quickly put me to sleep." At the same time she was taking four different medicines and occasionally she was "forgetting" to take those drugs prescribed for epilepsy.

"There was always the fight within myself that I could not and would not be an epileptic and that was the reason for my not taking my pills on a regular basis."

The headaches continued to be violent during her first marriage, which ended after six years. After the divorce, the headaches and seizures were fewer. Then a not uncommon post-divorce reaction took place.

"The fear of failing entered my life." It was not altogether relieved by her second marriage. "I married a successful man with two teenage children," she said. "I found myself falling into the same pattern as before—wanting to make him happy and pleased with me was my most important goal. This meant I would change my entire social life, my mode of dress (which had been changed for my first husband), and my manner. I did not feel all these changes were too much to ask, considering I was a willing subject all my life." But not all changes were so easy. "The most difficult seemed to be the frequent entertaining. It became essential to me, for each party given, to be absolutely perfect. My husband was and is a gourmet cook and belonged to a men's gourmet group. I had my work cut out, since I could, at that time, ruin baked potatoes.

"Fortunately and confidently, I can now say, after seven years of marriage we both shine in the kitchen. But, unfortunately, the more frequent the entertaining, the more headaches I would get."

Like many migraine victims, she tended to build a lot of stress into her life. "The stress of meeting people and worrying about meeting my husband's standards, fearing I would not be able to succeed at a high enough level in my own right so that he would be proud of me—all this created constant pressure. For the more I loved him, the more important it became to win a respect for me—a respect I unknowingly already had obtained."

As the years passed, a certain change took place in the headache pattern. "The violent migraines almost ceased," she said. "One would occur about every four months, lasting for a much shorter duration than in the past. The epileptic seizures decreased considerably—my husband made sure I took my medication. But during this time, everyday headaches became normal."

This was probably the time when the chronic daily headaches took command. "My husband did everything within his power to help alleviate my headaches. I was under the care of a prominent neurologist and a fine general practitioner. The following four years I spent some time with each of the following: a neurosurgeon, an internist, an allergist (when I had hives for four months), a Hapkido instructor (finger pressure), an osteopath, a chiropractor, and a physical therapist."

Somewhere, somehow, one would think she could have at least gotten relief from pain with such varied treatment. The cause of the headaches, the depression that seemed to have settled around her, might easily have been treated. But the cause of the depression—ah, that would have taken some very profound and skilled insight. Psychiatry is not my field, but I would venture to say that Anne Darby's depression was not caused by her marriage so much as by her sense of self—by her lifelong insecurities; by what she thought about herself, her life, and her adjustment to the pressures of both life and marriage. She expressed the pressures in this way: "Along with the insecurities I had acquired since childhood, there were the problems that were mounting with our combined children and my family."

She was taking up to 10 Excedrin a day for her headaches—far too many and too often—when suddenly another problem developed. "I took to my bed with a severe leg and back pain." It was diagnosed as a sciatic nerve problem. She also was losing weight—34 pounds in six months, a common indication of depression. Things really began piling up on her. She went to an orthopedic surgeon for her leg problems and had two violent leg spasms while in his office. She was admitted to a hospital, where she promptly had several epileptic seizures. Before they were over, she had four different doctors attending her, and she was undergoing everything from a spinal tap to an MRI to an electroencephalogram (EEG) in a search for everything from a brain tumor to epilepsy. Certainly there was no lack of effort on the part of medicine here. Yet nothing significant turned up on any test, though the EEG betrayed some irregularities (which might suggest epilepsy, among other things).

What followed was an incredible series of events in the hospital, which totally devastated Anne Darby.

"The first accident was falling out of bed with the rails up," she said. "I was so small that I fell through the two rails while reaching for a cigarette." (These days it may be hard for the reader to imagine that smoking was allowed in the hospital!) "They had neglected to tell me I had been given a sleeping pill along with my regular medication. Being quite dopey, I just climbed back into bed. But I attracted the attention of the floor nurses because I made quite a bit of noise knocking over my water pitcher and the telephone, which I'd been using to talk to a friend. I had hung up the phone without saying good-bye and went to sleep. They took me to X-ray without my remembering what happened after getting back into bed. The next morning my left eye was black.

"The following night they proceeded to tie me in to bed. I protested because one of my fears is to be held down or tied so I cannot move. My protesting was to no avail." (Fortunately, these days restraints such as these are only used as a last resort, with other methods of ensuring patient safety—such as having a nurse's aide assigned as a sitter in the room—tried first).

"Just as I was convincing myself it was for my own good and the sleeping pill would start to work very soon and it would be morning before I knew it and the ties would be off, the phone rang. Sure that it would be my husband and that his call would definitely make me feel better, I struggled to answer it. To my surprise and horror, it was an obscene phone call. The caller proceeded to tell me what he was going to do to me. I rang for a nurse again and was told to go to sleep. All I could think of was I was tied up and some man was going to come to my room and rape me and no one was going to help me."

"I'm not sure how much time passed, but I rang again. The head night nurse came. I was not believed when I told her of the call and was told outside calls could not come through the switchboard after hours. This definitely did not ease my mind. Now I was sure he was in the hospital waiting for the right time. I became hysterical and called my husband and father, insisting they come back to the hospital. After an hour of hysterical crying, my husband and father arrived with a private nurse and I was given a sedative. It was only after a psychiatrist took my case that they found out from the nurse's aide there actually had been an obscene phone call. The aide had gone off duty for a few days and neglected to report it."

"The next incident was to come while I was extremely ill. I had asked for a minister to stop by. A young chaplain, practicing his own philosophy instead of the work of God, arrived on the scene. During this time, each evening after hours, he proceeded to condemn, criticize, and interrogate me about my personal life until I refused to see him."

"After two weeks had passed, I began to have adverse reactions from the amount of medication that was given to me. My equilibrium was totally off; my hands would shake uncontrollably when I would lift them. The hospital staff searched my room for medication I might be taking on my own, but still they did not reduce the amount of medication they were giving me."

"I began to see things crawling at night, which must have been something like the DTs. I feel this was also due to the medication. The head night nurse was totally exasperated with me; she refused to leave a light on at night. So when a need to go to the bathroom late at night came, I did not want to upset the nurse by calling her. I proceeded to go by myself. On the way back, I passed out—or maybe I just fell, I'm not sure—into the corner of the nightstand, causing a great deal of damage to the right side of my face and ear."

Indeed, a few persons do suffer this as a side reaction to Dilantin, the anticonvulsive drug she was taking for epilepsy. "The next day," she went on, "I refused to take the Dilantin, sure that it was the cause of my shaking and loss of balance. Similar symptoms had occurred 10 years earlier with my first encounter with that medicine. I had informed the nurse of this just prior to the searching of my room.

"So, what started out as a sciatic nerve problem became a nervous breakdown—with a lot of help from people in the hospital to put me over the edge."

At this point, it was quite clear that she had urgent need of the psychiatrist. He did very well in his treatment. He not only settled her immediate anxieties but, as she later told me, "brought me a long way in understanding how to cope with my problems and insecurities. He also," she said, "made me aware that the mind can cause many illnesses in order to escape pressures you are not able to handle."

In the wake of all these events, her migraine had returned with terrible and violent force. Now the psychiatrist went to work on it. He succeeded in reducing it so that she was able to tolerate it. After two years, she said her more violent migraines were very few and her seizures—still considered as epileptic—were even fewer. They were down to nothing by the next year.

She was still getting headaches every day, however. She tried, as she had with migraine, not to let them dominate her life. "I went to great lengths to hide the fact I had a headache from my family and anyone else," she said. "Being a wife and mother has untold adventures, and constant pain dims those adventures." When the migraines diminished in force and frequency, she was so grateful that she felt that she could live with the daily headaches. But as time went on, she became anxious to rid herself of this pain also. "I wanted to see life as it really was to me, exciting and happy. Being tired and ill from the day-long pain, it was a struggle to keep up a front—to act like I really wanted to feel. I wanted to be cured."

One thing led to another: first to the beauty shop, then to a discussion of headache clinics and their work, and finally to my office in Chicago.

I gave her the customary tests. She certainly had migraine without aura which, thanks to the psychiatrist, was coming with considerably less violence (although with some force) than in the past. Her daily headaches were, I felt, chronic migraine, which most likely transformed due to long-term depression and made more difficult to treat due to medication overuse headache from Excedrin. (One clue that she was depressed: She'd awaken at 3 o'clock in the morning and, unable to get back to sleep, she would get up and pace the floor.)

Anne Darby was in need of inpatient treatment, but I knew this would be a difficult proposition for her given her awful experience with hospitalizations in the past. Together with our nursing staff, I explained to her our goals of inpatient treatment and why I felt this was absolutely necessary in her case. It would be very difficult for her to stop taking Excedrin daily without an increase in her daily headache pain levels for some time. The medications available at the Diamond Inpatient Unit would make that transition go much more smoothly. In addition, she would have the opportunity to learn a great deal about stress management through the classes and workshops offered. "Will you see me in the hospital, or will I be there 'on my own' with a bunch of doctors I've never met?" "Yes, I will see you every morning, and we will discuss how things have gone the day before, and I will keep you informed about the plan each and every day." With that, Anne Darby agreed to be admitted and arrangements were made for her to go to the inpatient unit that very afternoon.

I prescribed the antidepressant amitriptyline as a prevention medication for her headache. I explained that the drug would take some time before it began to improve her headache, but that it should begin to help her sleep even while she was in the hospital. We agreed that we would not judge its impact on headache for 3-4 weeks, well after she had returned home from the hospital.

But there was something more to be done. Anne Darby ultimately did not want to be on drugs. First, it was a visceral drive within her; second it was a conditioned drive from her hospital experiences. She'd been, as we've seen, on Dilantin, an anticonvulsant to control epilepsy, and she had experienced significant side effects from this. She was evaluated with an EEG during the hospitalization, and when this showed no irregularities, I suggested that she try to get along without it. She was delighted, all the more so because as time went by, she had no seizures. We discussed that, in the event her seizures may return,

131

we could try a newer antiepileptic drug which could also be very helpful for her headaches but would likely be better tolerated. For now she did not want to try any new daily medications besides the amitriptyline which we started during the hospital stay.

Anne Darby was very motivated to utilize nondrug treatment for her headache, and she embraced the biofeedback training during her hospital stay with great enthusiasm. It took two processes of training, of course. The "hot hands" technique to increase the flow of blood to the hands would take care of the migraine. The tone-relaxation technique to reduce the tension on the muscles in the head, face, and neck would take care of the tension headache. The training occurred for 20 minutes twice daily on each system in a special section at the Diamond Inpatient Unit.

We've already seen how biofeedback works in the treatment of migraine headaches. But there is another and distinctly different technique of biofeedback for the treatment of tension-type headache—especially those locked into depression or anxiety. It is based on research by Budzynski, Stoyva, and Adler of the University of Colorado. We know that much or all the pain in tension-type headaches is caused by a tightening of the muscles in the neck and in and around the head. The theory of biofeedback is that the patient can be taught to relax those muscles, and by relaxing them, to reduce or eliminate the pain.

The way we apply it at the Diamond Headache Clinic is to bring the patient into a quiet, dimly lit room and have him or her sit in a comfortable chair. The patient puts on earphones and has four electrically oriented leads attached to the forehead with tape. They are attached to the skin just over what we call the frontalis muscle. Generally, when the frontalis muscle relaxes, we find that so do the muscles of the scalp, neck, and upper body.

Of course, those leads are attached also to several electrical instruments. The instruments convert the tension into a graph that displays on

132

the computer screen in front of the patient, so that he or she can see the increase or decrease in muscle tension in real-time.

How does one learn to relax the frontalis muscle? By listening to a trainer repeating in low tones some thoughts that help induce relaxation. Here is an example of what one might hear and learn to say:

"Let all your muscles go loose and heavy. Just settle back quietly and comfortably. Wrinkle up your forehead now. Wrinkle and smooth it out. Picture the entire forehead and scalp becoming smoother as the relaxation increases. Now frown and crease your brows and study the tension. Let go of the tension. Smooth out the forehead once more. Now close your eyes tighter and tighter. Feel the tension. Now relax your eyes. Keep your eyes closed, gently, comfortably, and notice the relaxation. Now clench your jaws. Bite your teeth together. Study the tension throughout the jaws. Relax your jaws now. Let your lips part slightly. Appreciate the relaxation.

"Now press your tongue hard against the roof of your mouth. Look for the tension. All right, let your tongue return to the comfortable and relaxed position. Now purse your lips. Press our lips together tighter and tighter. Now relax the lips. Note the contrast between tension and relaxation. Feel the relaxation all over your face, all over your forehead and scalp. Eyes, jaws, lips, tongue, and your neck muscles. Press your head back as far as it can go and feel the tension in the neck. Roll it to the right and feel the tension shift. Now roll it to the left. Straighten your head and bring it forward and press your chin against your chest. Let your head return to a comfortable position, and study the relaxation. Let the relaxation develop.

"Shrug your shoulders. Right straight up. Hold the tension. Drop your shoulders and feel the relaxation. Feel how relaxed your neck and shoulders are. Shrug your shoulders again and mover them around. Feel the tension in your shoulders and in your upper back. Drop your shoulders once more and relax. Let the relaxation spread deep into your shoulders, right into your back muscles.

Relax your neck and throat, and your jaws and other facial areas as the pure relaxation takes over and grows deeper, deeper, ever deeper."

All of this takes only four or five minutes. But as the patient tenses his muscles, he sees the tension on the graph rise. As he relaxes them, he sees it go lower. Thus he learns that he can control the tension level on the graph simply by controlling the tension in these muscles.

Soon, he finds, he can lower the tension totally at will. Many patients reduce it significantly, and thus they achieve the near-total relaxation of the frontalis and accompanying muscles.

After several periods of practice, perhaps a week or two, the patient is able to relax the key muscles without the aid of the computer. He doesn't need to be hooked up to the electrical leads. He doesn't need to listen to the tone on the earphones. He simply exercises his ability to relax his muscles, and, in doing so, he reduces the pain that the taut muscles were causing.

Anne Darby, as we've seen, had to learn two biofeedback techniques— one for migraine headaches and the other for tension-type headaches. Yet she had no difficulty mastering them.

"After seven days in the hospital I went home, and after one week at home practicing 'bio,' everyday" she said, "I awoke for the first morning in years without a headache. My enthusiasm was almost uncontrollable." The more she tried it, the better it seemed. For she was not only controlling her headaches, she was controlling her life.

"Besides biofeedback, the classes on stress management and relaxation really helped me to learn to be less debilitated by stress and fear. Prior to this, I would have been in total agony, when entertaining, if the soufflé fell. Absolute disgrace," she said. "Now it is all chalked up to experience—failure is knowledge and people are a pleasant experience. The tension is under control. It is as if there's a warning bell ringing when it is time to practice being calm. For I have found the increased tension, pressure, and exasperation bring on not only tension headaches but the migraines.

"But calm is something I had never experienced. There is no one who can explain or tell you how to achieve inner calm, physician or otherwise. It must be experienced. Biofeedback was my guide to experience and relief."

In her enthusiasm, she became something of a missionary of biofeedback. It taught her a little more about human nature beyond anything that her ample experience might have suggested. "During my years with headaches," she told me, "I talked with many people about relief—where and how it might come about. Many of my fellow sufferers would say, 'If you ever find relief, be sure to let me know.' Then when I'd tell them about my relief through biofeedback, they were disbelieving. A lot of them seem to have little interest. Their typical comments would be 'I could not do that' or 'I am not going to get involved in anything like that' or 'I could not take the time'—these are the same women who are sometimes incapacitated for days because of migraine. It seemed as though they had excuses to avoid possible help. It makes one wonder how many need or want their condition."

Perhaps this was Anne Darby's most endearing quality. She wanted the help that medicine could give her.

16

THE TORMENTED ARTIST

My heart is an empty house.
Everything loved that lived there has gone long ago.
The scrambling and hurry of living has passed long ago.
The whispering and giggling of children,
Dog barking, the fuss of the aging,
Angry crying, bitter words, the purring of cats,
The rattling of feet, the telephone ringing ceased long ago.

I grieve to myself that ever this house should fall.

The paint will crack in the August sun
and weeds grow from the flagged steps;
Vines will push down through the roof
and rafters groan deep summer's rot,
For all these rooms are abandoned.
A spider will hang his lace from the stained lamps—
Float on his silver thread in the heavy dust,
Until winter howls through the doors
And icicles drip from the corniced shelves
For all these halls are abandoned.

I grieve to myself that his house will be forgotten.

And all that was built here, slowly, through the years
With infinite care and hope and love
Will vanish as though it had never been.

For the hardest stone will break,
For the heaviest wood will split,
Brilliant-hued glass will fade,
Printings and fine cloth powder.

Even the echoes of spirit voices dim into silence—
What has been done cannot be undone,
What is destroyed will not rise anew.
Sun and stars will whirl by in an endless sky.

I grieve to myself that ever this house must die.

At night while she slept, her right hand turned and reached out in an agonized twist. In the day her hours were filled with the nightmare of constant headache—"blurred vision, the feeling of constant pressure in the head." In the evening she had hallucinations—"ugly faces and whisperings. I tried to scream but I couldn't."

She had her own diagnosis: "I was afraid I was going bananas."

The first time that Lorraine Stelczyk came to our office, she had a haunted look in her eyes, a reminder of a problem unseen by others. The bones of her face were strong and prominent, a girdered structure holding together the folds of flesh. Her mouth was like a steel clamp. She was a relatively tall woman with a demeanor that communicated an air of regret for putting the world to the trouble of knowing her. Underneath all this restraint, this introversion, there was a personal vision of hell, a scream of anguish at the meaningless of human suffering. For Lorraine Stelczyk was a tormented person, terrified and directionless.

She was also one of the most remarkable women I've ever met. She was, and is, a gifted creative artist. She paints and she writes. The poem at the beginning of this chapter is hers. Her art is not soft pastel landscapes that echo

138

the whisper of spring rains; it is strong, macabre, grotesque, and it speaks of the canker that lies at the heart of our lives. It appeals, perhaps, to a special taste, yet the conception and the execution must one day, inevitably, I believe, earn her rank among the most accomplished artists of our time.

But Lorraine Stelczyk was not leading an artist's life. She was, for all intents and purposes, a suburban housewife. She'd been married for 12 years when I first met her. She lived in Hinsdale, Illinois, a most traditional suburb. She dressed neatly, but with a vague sense of the past tense, somewhat in the style of the antique dolls that she collected. She had no children, but she kept dogs; she loved to raise and show them. On the surface, she was, as she approached middle age, much closer—deliberately, I believe—to the style and traditions of the suburbs than to the life of a big city artistic community.

The reason she came to me was, of course, headache pain. She had a very severe migraine. Her headaches were coming on at an extraordinary rate— 8, 9, 10 times a month. Her headache condition had transformed to chronic migraine. The impact of this was almost continuous pain—in different parts of the head, to be sure, but with unremitting force.

This had gone on for years. In the last five months, the situation had become acute. She would as soon have given up breathing as given up painting, yet she had indeed given up painting. The pain was simply too great.

But her headaches were only the visible part of her problem. She was bothered by a great many other symptoms so intricate and intertwined that they all seemed to come together in a devastating crescendo. Rather than laying them out in clinical detail, I am relating them in a sort of stream-of-consciousness narrative as she expressed them over the weeks after she first came to our clinic:

"... some feeling of pressure in the head...couldn't see well enough to work...thing that bothered me most was the feeling of electricity in my head, like wires being pulled...had a dry mouth...wanted to eat more...did I want to get rid of the taste in my mouth? And yet as I began to feel better, I began to put more food on my plate...felt cold and sweaty at the same time...muscle

139

spasms...numbness...all once a week...hallucinations...two kinds...one was with the fan on in the basement and it was hot and I was dropping off to sleep...saw ugly faces...whispering...coming closer...the other was a woman's voice...heard it clearly...talking to me."

There were, to be sure, certain stresses and frustrations that had invaded her life. It had, she said, "taken me 15 years to get two degrees." She had gone to the Art Institute in Chicago, but, perhaps because of the style of her painting, her work had never been exhibited in a student show. ("I always had a lot of trouble in school.") Her marriage was a curious combination of dependencies. She provided, out of an inheritance, the financial basis of the marriage where her husband, who came to rely heavily on alcohol, provided the working details of the marriage. He would drive her wherever she needed to go, for example. "My mother was killed in an accident seven years ago. It was horrible. She lived for 11 hours..." She seemed to see a continuation of this somber event in what happened to her dogs: "One by one they died..."

All of this was manifested first through the migraine and then through chronic migraine and this brought her work to a stop. Here was a woman who was not able to cope—a woman who was not able to do the things that involved survival in the particular aesthetic as well as physical meaning that survival had for her.

Here also was a case that delineates dramatically the limits of success in treating headache. For I was going to attack the pain—successfully, but not overwhelmingly so. The treatment of Lorraine Stelczyk is the most explicit example of the highest, and most practical, hopes that a doctor can have in treating headache pain: to lift the patient out of complete helplessness and to get her back to the point where she can function again.

What I was not going to do was unravel all the intricate weavings of emotional and psychic tracings that underlined the life of Lorraine Stelczyk. To be sure, it is one phase of headache treatment to try to get at the cause of the pain after the pain has been muted. In many or most cases, this can be accomplished by letting the patient ventilate—by letting him tell you of the problem so that the patient himself becomes aware of it. But in very complicated cases, this is properly the function of a psychiatrist, not of a headache specialist. In such instances I will recommend, even urge, referral to a psychiatrist.

I remember one teenage boy who came to me for headaches and who, I could quickly see, was in deep emotional trouble. He was in a state that I recognized as pre-schizoid. Certainly, I could treat his headaches, but he needed other and more urgent treatment. I talked to other members of his family and, as best I could tell, they all needed psychiatric care. But the father was a hard-driving compulsive man who did not believe in psychiatrists. He would have none of it. So, I was faced with the problem of turning the boy away completely or of trying to help him in the best way I could, that is, in the treatment of his headache pain, and all the while hoping we could persuade the family to seek psychiatric help. It was a race against time, and it was a race we lost. One night I got a phone call from the police. The boy had broken every window in his home. It appeared that he had had a complete psychotic break. The police wisely took him to a hospital. By the time I got there, he was in a state in which all communication was impossible. The only person who could hope to treat him was a psychiatrist. Thus, the very treatment that his father denied him became the only treatment that could hopefully to reach the boy.

The case of Lorraine Stelczyk was not this severe. She was a bright and sensitive woman, and she would very likely seek psychiatric treatment at the moment she felt most in need of it. I did not feel that this was my role in treating her. My function was to lessen the pain in her head and help her return to a complete life.

There was another reason I was wary of playing the psychiatrist. I was aware that there is a conviction in some of the great creative artists that their torment is vital to their art. If you take their neuroses away from them, so the theory goes, you take away the roots of their creative drive and their art, whether it is writing or painting or performing, will decline or disappear. If Lorraine

141

Stelczyk had this apprehension, I was not going to invade her creative world by playing the part of psychiatrist until she asked for psychiatric help. My strategy was, as it is in so many cases of chronic migraine, to treat the depression and migraine at the same time. So, I prescribed one of the tricyclic antidepressants, amitriptyline (Elavil), and I suggested she return in two weeks.

In that time there was little change, which did not surprise me because on occasion, with the tricyclic antidepressants you do not get results that are immediate and overwhelming. It is a matter of blood levels and densities. Normally, I suggest waiting for a longer period before another visit in order to give the medicine a chance to take hold, but I wanted to see if something couldn't be done sooner for this woman, for I felt she was a lost soul.

So I had her return in another two weeks, just to examine and encourage her. I didn't want her to lose heart. For a lot of people *do* get discouraged; they take their medicine for two, three, or four doses, and then they drop it. When she returned for the second visit, her headaches were somewhat better. She said it was the first time she had gotten any kind of relief. She returned again in another two weeks and said that her headaches were "mild." There were numerous visits after that, and we adjusted her prescription up or down, depending on what she told us. But she came to believe, as we did, that we had her headaches under control.

Eventually, she went back to work. It was a joy in her life and a reward to mine, for it was an indication that we'd helped her become a functioning human being again. In fact, she came to my office one day and asked if I wouldn't want one of her paintings. I was enormously flattered. Her art gives depth and breadth to the human condition. It provokes thought as well as the emotions. But I didn't want to exploit her and I demurred. It didn't do any good. She came a few days later with one of her most treasured works. It hangs in my study today.

And yet, the treatment was not finished. Two years, or a little more, after we started, she came back and her headaches were significantly worse. It may have been because of the new stress in her life. She'd decided to get a divorce. As it turned out, the divorce was somewhat singular. For, although they lived apart, she continued to provide some financial help, when and if her former husband needed it. And if she needed help of a particular kind, he was there to provide it—he would still drop around to drive her wherever she needed to go.

So although there was no longer a love relationship, there was a working relationship, which both of them found useful and rewarding.

There was another possible reason for her problem. The tricyclic antidepressants sometimes lose their effectiveness in containing headache pain after a few years. Moreover, we had to mount the campaign against her migraine which was also present. So I switched her prescription from the tricyclic antidepressants to a monoamine oxidase (MAOI), a mood elevator that has proven to be very effective against migraine. But the MAOs require a little more time to become effective than do the antidepressants. Therefore, there is an interval of considerable pain between the time the antidepressants are discontinued and the MAOIs become effective. Why not use the antidepressants in tandem with the MAOs, to keep the pain minimal until the MAOIs become effective? Until the 1960s, many doctors used MAOIs in combination with antidepressants in treating depression, not headache. But treatments were found to go awry when these combinations were used. The reaction of the medical community was against the combination use of tricyclic antidepressants and MAOIs. In fact, it became a rule of medicine that a seven day period had to elapse between stopping one drug and starting the use of the other.

In recent years, however, these drugs are once again being used in combination, and without any indication of serious reactions. The change from previous practice is to select the patients more carefully and the dosages more probatively before using the combination. This is most conspicuously a field for the psychiatrist who is treating depression, it is an area of considerable controversy in medicine, and one which those of us in treatment of headache are

143

following very carefully. Studies at the Diamond Headache Clinic and other clinics have shown that the selective use of the tricyclic antidepressants, such as amitriptyline and doxepin, with MAOIs can be relatively safe.

In any case, we weaned Lorraine Stelczyk off the tricyclic antidepressants and started MAOIs with only a minimum of problems. She has control over her headaches once again and, with it, has control over her life. Her sleep is no longer disturbed by depression; she no longer has to spend hours or days in bed with migraine. She is working at her poetry and her painting, and more than that, she's added an important new dimension. She has learned that her work has value, that people want to buy it, so now she's letting it be exhibited at a few of the better shows in the nation, and she's letting it be purchased. Indeed, when people have expressed an interest in commissioning her work, she has listened and followed up on the opportunity. This was something she would not and *could* not do when she was bound by pain.

She is now 42 years old. She is not totally free of headaches. I did not cure her completely of them; I *could* not cure her altogether. But she is now a person who can not only survive but can cope and prosper at what she wants most to do.

Her style was suggested by the poem at the beginning of this chapter. Her range is suggested by the poem that follows. I offer it in the hope that you can begin to appreciate her as I do.

I lived with a yellow bird when I was young—
She put night away from me, rose with the sun.

She must have known monsters, the evil men do,
But locked fear up tight so that I never knew.

Rejoicing each hour in our sweet-flowered vine,
I forgot what must come with the passing of time.

144

And the blue-eye days ended,
Beasts come into their own,

I found her gold foliage
Torn red to the bone.

You bury a yellow bird
By the hedge with a knife,

But the music it made
You miss all of your life.

17

THE WOMAN WITH WHITE HANDS

She was small in stature, intelligent, somewhat driven, and forgetful.

When Geraldine Salter first came to me, she seemed like a perfect case. She'd had migraine headache since she was four years old. She was 36 now and the mother of three children. The headaches had been quite severe in the two years preceding her first visit with me. She'd get from two to four such headaches a month—one of them always during or just before her menstrual period and the other, she thought, at random times during the month, although I gradually came to understand that they were connected with ovulation.

Prior to an attack, she'd become crabby and high strung, which also is a sign of an oncoming menstrual period. She had no aura before an attack. She had severe nausea during an attack but no vomiting. Her hands felt cold, as they so often do in migraine. Her mother had migraine. Geraldine Salter's attacks seemed to increase when she was on birth control pills, which she'd been on the two years before coming to the Headache Clinic. The pain always attacked one side at a time, but it might come on one side in one headache, on the other side in another headache.

I've seen patients through their entire life having their migraines on only one side of their head. This generated the misconception held by many neurologists that one should look for an organic cause, like a brain tumor, in these patients. If it didn't, so went the theory, you must look for something organic. I remember one distinguished doctor who had migraine into his 40s. But it was not until then that the headache moved from one side of his head to the other. Until then, under the theory of the day, he was supposed to be suffering from something organic. He was, he later reported, enormously relieved when at the age of 40 he first suffered a migraine headache on the other side of his head. For that meant that he was not suffering from something

147

ominously malignant. Well, now we know that migraine can appear either way—locked always on one side of the head or moving from one side to the other.

It was apparent to me that Geraldine Salter did not have migraine with aura. (Some doctors believe that if a patient doesn't have an aura before the onset of pain, he doesn't have migraine. Now we know that 70 percent of the migraine victims do not get the aura. They have migraine, but not migraine with aura.) Geraldine Salter was virtually the perfect example of a person with migraine without aura. There was no mixture of headache pain, and there were no complications due to depression or anxiety. Therefore, we thought she was susceptible to very basic and direct treatment.

We started in the most basic and direct way possible by prescribing the use of a beta blocker. They had an early and significant impact on her headache pain, but they seemed to bother her tremendously in other ways. It was not altogether easy for her to articulate the condition because the symptoms seemed so elusive. But the most important element in them is that she seemed to feel that the coldness in her hands deepened when she took the medicine.

It was then that I discovered something she had forgotten to mention during her earlier visit. She had Raynaud's disease. This is a problem involving circulation of blood to the extremities. In her case, she felt an increasing coldness in her hands. Naturally, like most Raynaud victims, she was extremely sensitive to cold. In cold weather, her hands would turn very white, then a faint blue. The attacks, in this case, would come and go, leaving the patient in considerable discomfort, but in no particular danger. (If ignored and allowed to progress, however, Raynaud's disease may lead to gangrene.)

With the belated information about her having Raynaud's disease, we were able to prescribe another medicine that would not affect the blood vessels in her hands. It was phenelzine (Nardil), the monoamine oxidase inhibitor (MAOI)—a mood-elevator which, as we've seen, has been proven effective against migraine. It proved effective in this case. Geraldine Salter's headache came quickly under control, and in a month or so it began to diminish and then to disappear.[4]

But again, here was an opportunity, and an almost ideal one, to take the patient off drugs. Biofeedback would help treat both her migraine and her Raynaud's disease. You'll recall how it works in the case of migraine: The patient is trained to decrease the flow of blood through the swollen blood vessels of the head and increase the flow of blood to the hands, thus reducing the pain of migraine. The way the patient knows that the training is working is by the increased temperature of the hands. By thinking of the hands getting increasingly warmer and then hotter, the individual is able to raise the temperature of the hands and, by the achievement, increase the flow of blood through them.

Geraldine Salter proved very adaptable to the disciplines of biofeedback. She mastered the technique swiftly and was readily able to raise the temperature of her hands. Indeed, she became so accomplished at it that she became a model for the technique when demonstrations were held at medical meetings. She was able to attack the migraine by noticing when she felt particularly high-strung or crabby. Just sitting down in a quiet room and concentrating—part of the discipline of biofeedback—helped relieve her of those symptoms, and the change in flow of blood helped relieve her of headache pain. More than that, it helped her overcome the impact of Raynaud's disease.

The lesson is an important one for doctor and patient. For the doctor: Keep exploring the past history of the patient to determine other factors implicated in the headaches or its treatment. And for the patient: Don't forget the details of anything that's happened to you when talking with the doctor.

---

[4] See Appendix II, Drugs Used in Acute Migraine Attacks

18

THE STUDENT WHO COULDN'T STUDY

Some people might describe Erin Donnelly as the all-American teenager. That might be an old-fashioned term, but this bright, pretty 17-year-old girl from a tiny town in Iowa truly personified this somewhat outdated way of looking at youth. She was not only a top athlete (she was a member of her high school's cheerleading squad and gymnastics team) but she was also a straight-A student. In fact, she was absolutely thrilled that she was going to be attending a Big Ten school—The University of Wisconsin—in the fall. She planned to study veterinary medicine. All in all, everything was going extremely well for Erin Donnelly—everything, that is, except the headaches.

The onset of the headaches had been rather sudden. They started during her last term in high school. However, once she got that first headache, she began to suffer the same severe, incapacitating pain on a daily basis. And with these headaches, came some very noticeable personality changes. She started having difficulty sleeping, concentrating, and basically doing anything she had done before her headaches started. She found little enjoyment in that activities that had once been so exciting and had given her so much joy. But just as important to this conscientious teenager was the fact that her schoolwork was suffering as a result of her headaches. She received mostly Bs and Cs that last term. She simply could not study with the intense, constant pain in her head.

During the summer, Erin Donnelly and her parents tried to find some help for her pain. They went to see many doctors who prescribed many different medicines and methods of relief for her headaches. She even tried acupuncture. Although some of the drugs provided modest relief, none proved to be a solution to the daily occurrence of the headaches. The relief, in most instances, was short-lived.

Despite her daily pain, she began college in the fall. But she found that she had difficulty keeping up with her classes because of poor concentration. She also had no social life in spite of her normally perky personality and youthful good looks. Erin Donnelly really had lost any interest she may have had in going out and being social. She had become preoccupied with her pain and seriously considered dropping out of school. She went to the Student Health Service one day to get something for the pain and was referred to the Diamond Headache Clinic.

She came to her first visit at the Clinic with her parents. They were obviously concerned and were very supportive and loving. There was absolutely no evidence of rebellion on her part or of anger between Erin Donnelly and her parents, yet the young woman was quite obviously depressed and flat. The reason I was so concerned about her relationship with her parents is that you often see young adults with depression that is precipitated by feelings of rebellion and anger within the family. This was clearly not the problem in this case. I then decided to probe deeper into the exact time the headaches began. She and her parents noted that the headaches and subsequent behavioral changes had been a recent occurrence, only during the past six months or so—"just after the accident."

"What accident," I asked rather excitedly.

"I was in a minor car accident with my boyfriend," She replied. "It was really nothing. No one was hurt, really, and the car had only minor damage."

"Was your car hit from behind?" I asked.

"Yes, as a matter of fact," she said. "I bumped my head on the dashboard, but I was checked buy a doctor, underwent a barrage of tests, and was declared perfectly fine. I didn't have any cuts or bruises, just a stiff, sore neck."

"And the headaches?" I continued.

152

"They started about two days after the accident," she replied. That was the key. I knew what Erin Donnelly was suffering from—she had "posttraumatic" syndrome.

The posttraumatic syndrome can include a variety of different symptoms—headaches, mood disturbances, difficulty in concentrating, insomnia, irritability, and so on. (Erin Donnelly, you will recall, exhibited many of these symptoms, not just the headaches.) The posttraumatic headache does not have any specific characteristics except that the pain has been preceded by an injury. The headaches and other symptoms can continue for many years after the injury occurs. These symptoms usually develop within 24 to 48 hours following trauma, although at times there may be a more delayed onset.

Posttraumatic headache can mimic almost any type of chronic, recurring headache. It may be constant or intermittent and may involve any areas of the head or even the entire head. Dr. Harold G. Wolff, the noted headache researcher, divided posttraumatic headache into three primary groups. The first group resembles tension-type headache. The second type is caused by scar tissue from the injury, and the third is a vascular headache, like migraine—one-sided, with nausea, vomiting, and swelling of the arteries of the scalp. Furthermore, tension-type and vascular (migraine) headaches may occur simultaneously, and the term *posttraumatic headache* may describe this combination.

Management of posttraumatic headache depends on the mechanism responsible for the headache. Those headaches resembling tension-type headaches respond best to tricyclic compounds, such as amitriptyline, imipramine, and doxepin. The chronic migraine headaches should be treated similarly, but with the addition of a beta blocker, such as propranolol. Moreover, biofeedback, using the techniques of general body relaxation, specific muscle relaxation, and hand-warming, may be quite useful, particularly in combination with these medications. Those headaches that fall into the vascular (migraine) category should be managed exactly like a nontraumatic migraine. They may respond to a combination of tricyclic compounds and beta blockers, but other medication, such as cyproheptadine, clonidine, or calcium channel blockers may be beneficial. In addition to the aforementioned medications and biofeedback, it is also vital to address the psychological factors in many of these patients, where these factors appear to be playing an important role in the continuation of the chronic headache or other posttraumatic symptoms. Posttraumatic headache and the other related symptoms have an impact not only on the patient but also on the patient's family, employer, friends, and others. Not only are there emotional symptoms resulting from organic disturbances produced by the head injury, but powerful forces enhancing these symptoms are generated by the continued head pain, impaired memory, loss of concentration, and so forth. This combination can create an ideal setup for a cyclical effect.

Thus, the most appropriate management of the posttraumatic headache involves consideration of all these factors as well as pharmacotherapy, biofeedback, and the usual modes of psychotherapy.

Because of the severe, incapacitating nature of Erin Donnelly's headaches, I felt hospitalization in our inpatient headache unit at Presence/Saint Joseph Hospital would be beneficial. My goal was to decrease the amount, severity, and duration of her headaches; to stabilize her on a medication regimen; and to manage her pain with the use of simple, non-narcotic analgesics within acceptable limits. I also ordered the usual tests, including an MRI, so I could rule out the possibility that an abnormal lesion or mass was causing her headaches. I treated her with an MAOI, an NSAID, and a tricyclic antidepressant. Within three days, she was sleeping well, her mood was dramatically improved, and her headaches were diminished substantially. I released her from the inpatient headache unit after a five-day stay. Her headaches have remained under excellent control since her discharge from the hospital more than nine months ago.

Erin Donnelly is now busily involved in dorm activities and an exciting, fun-filled social life at the University of Wisconsin. Moreover, I'm very happy to say that she received three As and one B after her first college semester.

19

THE WOMAN WHO HATED TO STAND UP

When I walked into the examination room, the patient was lying down on the table.

"I'd rather talk to you lying down, doctor," she said.

"No trouble," I said. "Just lie there and relax."

In the next few minutes, she told me some of the highlights of her case. She was 45 years old and the mother of five children. She'd begun getting very intense headaches two or three weeks earlier. There was no explanation for them, but the pain was unbearable whenever she stood up. When the attacks came on, she had to lie down, it was the only relief she could get. The over-the-counter headache remedies didn't make a dent on the mask of pain.

She was a tall woman, German in ancestry, stoic in temperament. When she conceded that the pain was bad, you had to believe that it was very bad. It became worse when she got up and moved around. Indeed, it must have been torture for her even to come to the office.

Cautiously, I explored the possibility that it was a migraine headache. She had some of the migraine signs: the desire to lie down, the tendency toward nausea and vomiting, and the inclination toward vertigo. But she had no aura and she did not have migraine personality. It seemed unlikely that migraine would have struck a woman of middle age so suddenly, coming on with such a maddening rush that within two weeks she'd be seeking medical help.

She did exhibit some of the stiffness of the neck that we often associate with tension-type headaches. There was certainly a great deal of stress in her life. For example, she was a Roman Catholic, yet, despite the disciplines of her church, she'd been married twice. Moreover, her first husband, then 25, had left her to marry a 54-year-old woman. I suggested that she be admitted to the hospital so we could take a more thorough look at her. "I think we can help

157

you," I assured her. She agreed, and the MRI of her brain was normal. We did a lumbar puncture (spinal tap) and measured the pressure of the fluid in her spinal column, which was less than half of what it should have been, and the origin for such spinal fluid is in the brain.

The reasons for a lowering of the pressure in the spinal column are many. It may be due to surgery on the cranium or on the spinal column. It may be due to some sort of significant injury, or it may come on spontaneously, as it seemed to have done in this case. (There is a theory that in apparently spontaneous onsets there has been a seemingly insignificant incident that the patient has forgotten, perhaps a fall or a strain of some sort.) The condition was easily corrected. We simply injected a fluid into the spinal column that raised the pressure to normal. Her headaches disappeared almost immediately.

But I was concerned about another problem that lingered in my memory. At a medical meeting, we'd examined six cases in which the patients had low spinal pressure. On further examination, four of the patients had blood clots in the cranium.

In recent years, a very easy procedure has been perfected. It's called an MRA, like an MRI but with injecting a dye, and it visualizes the circulation of the brain in an easy diagnostic way. The MRA revealed something significant. It was a small blood clot on one side of her head. We took a close look again and found a small blood clot on the other side of the head.

She was referred to a neurosurgeon who scheduled the patient for a surgical procedure. The surgery involved boring holes in the cranium about the size of a nickel, then opening the membrane over the brain so the clots were exposed. Then a rubber tube was inserted into each hole and the matter causing the blood clots was sucked out very gently. The wounds were closed and she was sent to the recovery room.

In this case, the patient recovered completely and without complications. She was discharged from the hospital on the eighth day she'd been there. She was, and is, completely free of headaches or any other symptoms of problems in the spine or brain.

Her case had a beneficial aftereffect. It taught the neurosurgeon and me something about the process of this disease. We learned that the disease has its own disguise; it does not show anything in neurological exams or MRIs. The symptom is the clue. The headache-when-standing-up is a powerful indication of what is wrong. The neurosurgeon in this case later told me that, although he'd never remembered a case quite like this before, he had five of them that he immediately recognized and diagnosed during the next year.

20

THE MISPLACED MIGRAINE

One of the dangers of writing about headache pain in a way that tempts the reader to find himself or herself in these cases, is that there are so many cases that are not typical. These are cases where the totally unpredictable has taken place. They tend, in a doctor's workload, to be memorable. For the patient and the reader, they serve as warnings that there is very little in medicine that can be said to happen the same way all the time. It is in these variations from the norm that we find some of the mystery, excitement, and frustration of medicine.

The case of Marcie Dolan is an example. She was an intense young woman, piquant of feature, slight of build, sharp of mind, and intense in her view of herself. When she would visit the Clinic, she'd have a long list of questions all drawn up, and she wanted the answers. The central cause of this was her intense and quite frequent headache pain. By the time I first saw her, she was having excruciating headaches as often as two or three times a week. Naturally, any person in this kind of pain might suffer severe tests of emotional equilibrium—particularly when you understand she's undergoing other tests of mind and body, such as pregnancies. Any person in this kind of pain is powerfully motivated to seek escape from it.

The mystery was not in what kind of headache she had, it was migraine, but rather in why it was not recognized and treated before she came to our clinic. There were plenty of clues: her mother, grandmother, and great-grandmother had migraine, and there is some indication that her daughter also had it. The early headaches appeared to come in conjunction with her period, she got blurred vision in association with the pain, and, as is typical in migraine, she got the headaches on one side of her head—in her case, the right side.

But there was one significant difference. She got the headaches in the back of her head instead of in the front, over or behind one eye or the other. And it was that inconsistency, that single variation from the norm, that perhaps caused so much of the problem. If only because it could not be fully explained, her headache became the center of the problems that were building up around her.

"Unlike my mother and my daughter," said Marcie Dolan, "I never had any headaches that I can remember as a child or a teenager. I began to experience headaches only when my first child was about 18 months old. My only previous health problem had been some severe stomach pains, for which the doctor prescribed a mild tranquilizer. My second pregnancy, which followed shortly after, appeared to trigger more frequent migraines." That was, of course, unusual. Migraine pain tends to disappear during pregnancy because of the change in the hormonal balance of the body.

Soon she noticed a dramatic change in her energy level. She developed an almost compulsive need to get things done. "On the day preceding the migraine," she said, "my energy level was always extremely high." This is not altogether unusual in migraine victims. I've had a good many patients who experience a soaring sense of energy before or after their migraine. People may get several days of housework done in a matter of two or three hours. Those who also work outside the home may pour themselves into whatever physical or mental labor is available and accomplish goals that might have taken them days or weeks in other periods.

Unfortunately, Marcie Dolan also began to experience other symptoms. One of them was vertigo, "which fluctuated in severity according to my monthly cycle." She went to the doctor, and he gave her a series of tests that "showed nothing more than a thyroid functioning at above-average levels." When the vertigo disappeared, she attributed it to her third pregnancy. Unfortunately, her migraine increased in frequency and intensity. "This totally amazed my mother," she said, "because in the 50 years that she suffered from migraine, she was completely free from them only during her two pregnancies."

When Marcie Dolan's third baby was born, the migraine reverted to a once-a-month pattern, but the vertigo returned. It began to distress her and her family. "I was sent to numerous specialists and underwent many tests," she said. She found greater solace in the report of a chiropractor: he said he'd spotted a pinched nerve at the base of her skull.

In all of this, you can see that the pain was beginning to dominate her life and even that of her family. When she became pregnant again, for the fourth time, the migraine headaches increased once again. Now they began appearing three times a week, "each lasting approximately 24 hours." Only if you've had a severe migraine can you appreciate how devastating this is to the life and composure of the victim. It means that half of every week is going to be spent in a pain from which there is no escape and for which there is no adequate explanation.

Once again the headaches abated after the baby was born and became a once-a-month phenomenon. For a long while, nothing seemed to alter that pattern. "Regardless of what pressure or tension I would be under, I never had migraine more than once a month," she said. In time, the pace and pattern of her headaches changed. "At about the time I reached the age of 30, I became plagued by some very intense headaches that did not follow the normal migraine pattern," she said. For a while each month, she'd get headaches almost daily— "headaches that created the feeling of a pressure exploding all over my head. The pain was almost more excruciating than that of the sharp, throbbing pains of migraine." Then the headaches would go away as suddenly as they came: "One morning I would awaken and my head would be completely clear of any pain or pressure. I felt fantastic! All was fine for several days until my routine migraine would come on for the month. Then the entire cycle would repeat itself."

There were indications that some of the headaches she felt had something to do with hormonal changes in her body. That might have made them another variation of her migraine "Now I suffered from extreme fatigue that a few months later was determined to be caused by a thyroid gland

163

functioning considerably below average." You recall that several years earlier the vertigo had been attributed to an overactive thyroid. Now she feels that the low thyroid activity, called hypothyroidism, will be with her for most of the rest of her life. "Hypothyroidism is an inherited trait from father's side of the family," she explained. But there is ample medication to control the problem, and she saw consolation in all this. "The headaches decreased even more, and I felt great."

The headaches were not gone; they were merely reduced and regular in nature. "I found myself on a cycle whereby I could expect a 48-hour migraine every three weeks, to the day," she said.

The weeks stretched into months and the months into years. She was regular in her cycle of migraine, and yet she was not deeply tormented by it. She'd learned how to adjust to it. There is a fortitude in this, and perhaps even a nobility. There are not many among us who would accept stoically the knowledge that we are going to suffer very intense pain for 48 hours every three weeks, and not shrink before that knowledge. There is something to be said for the mettle and the intrepid nature of the migraine victim—something that we might wish for ourselves in our moments of trial.

Everything remained regular and unwavering with Marcie Dolan until just four years from the time she was diagnosed with depression. "Then, rather suddenly, the migraine headaches again increased in both frequency and severity," she said. "Each headache lasted three days, with just a one-day break before a new one would start up again." The pain was so great that she began taking powerful painkillers as well as over-the-counter remedies: "I was taking one Norco (hydrocodone) along with two Excedrin every $2^{1/2}$ to 3 hours." They had little effect on the headaches. "This," she said, "is when I began seeking help in earnest."

She went to an internist, who prescribed a tranquilizer and urged her to enter the psychiatric ward of a local hospital. She went to her family doctor, who disagreed with the need for the tranquilizer and took her off all medication. "He felt that many of my headaches were induced by a hormone imbalance," she said. He, too, recommended that she go into a hospital, and get an MRI. There was no clue as to the source of her migraine, but while in the hospital, she suffered a recurrence of the "pressure" headaches. Her family doctor called in a gynecologist and a neurologist as consultants.

The gynecologist decided that she'd begun to develop an ovarian cyst. He prescribed medication, "And within several days the pressure headaches again ceased."

The neurologist prescribed several medicines, one after another, as he sought to find something that would reduce her migraines. One of them was an anticonvulsant, which caused, she said, a severe personality change which greatly alarmed her and also produced an allergic reaction so that she needed further medication to offset the personality change and the allergic rash. Her confidence was beginning to waver and it lowered when the neurologist advised her to see a psychiatrist. The psychiatrist promptly reported back to the neurologist that her emotions were stable and that they did not appear to trigger the migraine headaches.

It was then that the neurologist recommended that her occipital nerve be cut or neutralized with alcohol injections. That is a nerve leading to the key portion of the back of the head. Some doctors, not recognizing the migraine possibilities in the region, decide that the pain is something known as "occipital neuralgia" and that it can be treated by deadening the nerve leading to the region. I see cases every week or two in which the occipital nerve has been severed or otherwise treated, and the tragedy is that it is so often a useless form of surgery.

Fortunately, Marcie Dolan reacted against having it done. For one thing, it threw her into a state of panic, for another, the family doctor was against it. He felt that the headaches might better be treated through medication than surgery. And finally, her family was against having it done. So now she was at the end of the road. She had the headache, she had many doctors, she had an ultimate choice, which she did not like.

I recognized that she had a migraine headache, even if it was attacking in the back of her head. I also recognized that we had to work within the legitimate dimensions of her medication. She had an underactive thyroid; I was not about to take her off the medication for that problem. She was taking hormones to offset the aftereffects of a hysterectomy (and to give her confidence that the pressure headaches would not return). As we have discussed, the addition of estrogen can worsen or improve a patient's migraine condition, or it may have no impact whatsoever. There is no way to predict which will occur, however. In Marcie Dolan's case, I felt the addition had indeed worsened her headache condition. At my urging, she gave up her hormones for several weeks. Then she told me, quite candidly, that she felt that she needed them. I acceded to her request. First, I prescribed a beta blocker—propranolol. Then I followed up with an antiepileptic drug, topiramate. Bit by bit, this seemed to get the headaches under control.

Finally, I introduced her to biofeedback. It would allow her to get off the antimigraine drugs, which, considering that she had other medications to consume, would be helpful. As it turned out, she responded beautifully to biofeedback, mastering the technique and keeping her headaches well under control.

It was, of course, a biofeedback program for migraine. For even though it struck in an unusual place and at an unusual tempo, it was this most difficult and apparent of headaches. It has been my experience that many difficult cases where there is a multitude of psychological problems respond well to the relaxation exercises of biofeedback.

Right now, I expect that Marcie Dolan is in her home, which is about 100 miles from my office, writing down questions she plans to ask at her next visit. I can't blame her. For it took a long time and a lot of difficult treatment to get down to the questions that counted: "I've got a migraine. People tell me it

166

can't be a migraine because it isn't where migraine normally appears. Is it possible that it's a migraine that's been misplaced? And if so, can it be treated?"

The answers to those last two questions turned out, eventually, to be yes.

21

THE WOMAN WITH THE SECOND CHANCE

I remember the first time I saw Fran Carson. It was 1981, and she had come to the Headache Clinic from her home in the Southwest seeking help for the "intense, piercing" in her head, a pain she had suffered for nine long years. Her headache problem was not particularly difficult to diagnose. She was suffering from migraine with aura. Her pain was one-sided and was always preceded by an aura or warning that the pain was on its way. In her particular case, she saw "sparkles." I also suspected, and later confirmed, that Fran Carson was suffering from tension-type headaches as well. She shared some intimate details about her family life—details that obviously were causing her a fair amount of stress. This stress was likely to be the precipitating factor in her tension-type headaches. Her first marriage had been painful and eventually—some 25 years later—resulted in a traumatic divorce. Her first husband, a heavy drinker, had been both mentally and physically abusive. Her second marriage was another story. She had married a wonderful and caring man. Yet it was obvious that she was still carrying around a lot of pent up anger and hostility from that first marriage. She also revealed that she had been deeply hurt by her eldest daughter and that their relationship was shattered beyond repair. Her frank and open revelations about her personal relationships made my diagnosis easy. Unfortunately, things aren't always as simple as they seem.

During that first visit, I also discovered that her previous physician had prescribed a triptan to try and help Fran Carson with her headache problem. This drug is commonly used to abort an acute attack of migraine and is considered effective and safe in recommended doses. I suspected that she was exceeding the recommended use and that worried me in light of her age. Excessive use of triptans can lead to rebound headaches. During the 1970s, P.P.H. Humphrey and his team of researchers at Glaxo in the United Kingdom attempted to identify the serotonin receptor types responsible for the beneficial effects of serotonin in headache. They identified a serotonin receptor type 5-HT1B, which is mainly found in the cranial blood vessels rather than in the peripheral blood vessels. Because of this discovery, the scientists were able to design agonists that could stimulate the receptors and trigger constriction of the cranial blood vessels and help terminate an acute migraine attack. This was a much more effective treatment than ergotomine, but had similar consequences with its daily use. In 1988, they utilized a serotonin (5HT)(1B/ID) agonist called sumatriptan, to treat migraine and certain other headaches. Many pharmaceutical companies developed similar drugs as effective as sumatriptan, and they were called triptans. The triptans act by binding two serotonin receptors in the brain, which leads to a reversal of blood vessel swelling. Sumatriptan was approved by the U.S. Food and Drug Administration (FDA) and became available by prescription in 1992. Eventually other triptans were approved and were available in a variety of forms for administration, including oral, intranasal, and transdermal. Fran Carson was 57 years old when she came to see me. Although she wasn't taking the triptan every day, at least not yet, she was clearly on a path of self-destruction, one that needed immediate attention. I advised her that I wouldn't be able to tackle her headache problem until she could get her triptan problem under control, and I told her I would help her with it. I urged her to enter the hospital so that we could help her break the rebound headache cycle. She said she would think about it and get back to me before she left Chicago the next day. I left the office that night hoping she would call because I was truly afraid that she wouldn't get a second chance. I waited for her call the next day, but it never came.

Sumatriptan quickly became the most consistently effective treatment for acute migraine headache. It also has the most prolonged effect. However, it must be taken with care, in moderations, and only by those migraine sufferers who can tolerate this powerful drug. It shouldn't be taken by children, by patients with circulatory or cardiac problems, or by pregnant women. Some of its effects are nausea, vomiting, diarrhea, numbness or tingling in the arms or legs, coldness or pallor in the hands and feet, leg cramps or weakness, and chest pain. Moreover, sumatriptan should not be taken on a daily basis or patients may suffer from rebound headaches. In this situation, they continue to take the sumatriptan on a daily basis because it relieves the headaches. The patients then build a tolerance to the medication and start taking increasing amounts of the drug. Eventually, the sumatriptan itself will cause the headaches. It is very difficult to treat those patients until they have stopped taking the triptan. I was afraid that this rebound phenomenon would begin to affect Fran Carson if I didn't try to help her beat the triptan habituation. More importantly, I was afraid of the ultimate consequence she would likely face as a result of her continued overuse of the drug—the possible shortening of her life.

It took six years, but Fran Carson eventually called. She told me that she was ready to deal with her habituation and her headache problem. She flew to Chicago immediately and I admitted her to the Clinic's inpatient headache unit at Presence-Saint Joseph Hospital. It was a difficult withdrawal. People who are triptan- habituated are probably the most difficult patients to treat, because the addiction is not a true psychological addiction, but rather it is a physiological addiction. The body becomes accustomed to the triptan. Fran Carson's detoxification took about 10 days. I was greatly surprised to see that the triptan had not caused any coronary damage, despite the fact that she had been taking the drug every day for many, many months. It was a clear and simple fact: Fran Carson had been extremely lucky. With her drug habituation under control, I was then able to tackle her headache problem. We treated her with a beta blocker, an NSAID, and a non-narcotic analgesic. This combination has been very effective in reducing her migraine attacks as well as her tension-type headaches. At last report, Fran Carson said she was relatively headache-free— she gets a moderate headache every month or two but that's all. She never told me what finally motivated her to return to the Clinic more than six years after that first visit. Whatever the reason, it was gratifying to know that she had taken charge of her life, essentially giving herself a second chance at living a pain-free existence.

22

THE $250,000 HEADACHE

One of the great truisms of our time is that stereotypes fail in our minds, just as they do in our society. The same is true in medicine, including headache medicine. Since migraine is much more common in females, and since migraine is the most common headache condition for which a person will seek medical treatment, most headache patients treated by physicians tend to be female. So if one thinks of the "typical" headache patient, one probably envisions a female. That assumption is, of course, often not accurate.

Chip Tewelk was such an example: he was male, young, very strong, and athletic, yet he had severe and prolonged headaches, and he was in a clinical depression. What he did not seem to realize, however, was the degree to which the two conditions were related.

One of the tip-offs is that he associated his headache as beginning with a particular accident. This happens with victims of chronic posttraumatic headache. Patients with chronic posttraumatic headache are at increased risk of depression. In some migraine patients, head trauma can change the headache frequency and severity rather significantly.

"In 2007," said Chip Tewelk, "I received a head injury during a high school football game. The blow was to the front of the head after running head-on into one of my own players. I do not remember how long I was 'out,' but I remember being carried off the field." He was checked by a doctor at the game, and later he had a CT scan at a hospital. No injury appeared, but he began to have headaches within one week. He was given the OK to play again a week later. At the time, it was not only his head that pained him, but also a soreness in his middle and lower back. But it was the head that he was to have an enduring concern about: "In 2009, I was knocked out again playing football and once again the in the fall of 2010. I had headaches nearly every day since that first hit."

Physically, Chip Tewelk violated every notion of the depression stereotype. He was a stocky, strong youth; he weighed 191 pounds and, as a weight lifter, he was able to lift more than $2\frac{1}{2}$ times his own weight, a formidable physical achievement. Like many athletes, he also had an awareness of himself, of his fine physical condition, and of any deviation from it. "The other odd physical behavior came during the wrestling season in 2009," he said. "I began to fatigue easily during matches and would often have a hard time leaving the mat after a match. But I do not know if this was psychological or physiological."

Like many teenagers, Chip Tewelk had reacted dramatically to any change from the status quo—any change that might become a focus of discontent. "I became very depressed in the fall of 2009 because of my performance in football," he related. "I had made it my life, and I was not satisfied with it." In seeking to explain this disappointment to himself, most of all, he searched for outside factors. One was his glasses. "I blamed it on the burning of my contact lenses because I had a poor fit. I was disgruntled, to say the least." Another was his social relationships. "I got messed up with a girl, and one mistake after another popped up." All these things had a lowering impact on him. "My expectations were not reached, and I made myself suffer for it." In retrospect—from the perspective of many years and considerable treatment he is aware now of what might have been happening to him then. "Now I see I was entering possibly into mild depression."

In 2010, he entered college: the Citadel, a military-oriented college of the liberal arts on the outskirts of Charleston, South Carolina. Like a good many youngsters, he found it difficult to make the adjustment to college, particularly in a college of rather unwavering traditions and stringent discipline. "I was definitely not prepared for what was to take place for the next nine months," he said. "The atmosphere in the school was rigid, and I was not ready for it." It was

174

not so much the studies but the demeanor required of the students—the stand-at-attention-with-neck-braced position common, say, to plebes at other military colleges such as West Point. "During these nine months, it was like I was in hell from the constant bracing," he continued. He felt his scalp was contracting and the only relief he would get was "hitting someone head-on in football practice."

He became increasingly tense and nervous, and he began getting more severe headaches. The headaches might naturally have followed an increasing depression and so might a stiff neck. He attributed it to the "bracing" stand-at-attention that he had to maintain most of the day. But the feeling of stiffness or rigidity in the neck is a characteristic often seen in persons suffering from a chronic depression. "The last three weeks at school," he said, "I stayed in the infirmary."

When the headaches continued that summer, he entered a hospital for a battery of neurological tests including an MRI and, and an electroencephalogram (EEG). "Everything was normal except the EEG," he said. "The doctor called it a seizure disorder. Of course, this scared me to death." The doctor prescribed an anticonvulsant drug. It was a drug that is often the first choice of neurologists when they feel they're treating a migraine headache. He then suggested that Chip Tewelk see a psychiatrist. "This also scared me."

He went to a psychiatrist about the headaches and then an ophthalmologist, an allergist, an oral specialist, and a number of general practitioners. Still the headaches persisted.

"I enrolled at a local college but quit after a few days because of the pain in my eyes and the front top of my head, along with the pulling in my neck." He went through a long winter like this and then suggested to his parents that he seek further psychiatric help in an effort to overcome the pains in his head.

This time he enrolled at a famous university clinic in the Southeast. He underwent hypnosis and he worked his way through a large number of psychological tests. "I came back no better off than before," he said.

Nevertheless, he continued to take a number of medicines that the doctors in the clinic recommended. They involved everything from tranquilizers to selective serotonin repute inhibitors (SSRIs), including sertraline and fluoxetine—drugs that combat the changes in the chemicals around the brain during migraine. "I took these for about three months and then flushed all of them down the toilet," he said. "None of my symptoms stopped—the burning headaches in the front and top of my head."

Yet he tried to resume life in its normal tempo. He went back to college. He worked at a camp for the blind. ("I thought the answer would come about if I tried to give instead of receive.") He threw himself into weight lifting. "As usual," he said, "I was obsessed to be the best. I once lifted 525 pounds in the dead lift. This would strain anybody, but I had it in my head to do it. I strained myself every day, but I would not listen to my body." And still the headaches came and persisted until he was driven once again to seek the help of a psychiatrist. He fled the psychiatric help once again: "I became worse and did not return to school in the fall."

Instead, he went back to a hospital and had another whole series of tests run—tests identical to those run in the same hospital a year or so earlier. The results were the same as those of a year earlier: Everything was normal except his EEG. "This still scared me," he said. He was seeing a neurologist, who sent him to an eye, ear, nose, and throat specialist. The specialist treated him for polyps on his sinuses, for suspected allergies, and for hypoglycemia (lower-than-normal blood sugar content, which he treated with vitamin shots and a special diet). To this were added treatments with cortisone and histamine. "None of these worked either," he said.

It had been six years since the head injury he first remembered. Now he just surrendered to pain. "This whole school year (2013-2014) I sat around the house in an apathetic condition," he said. "I did not do anything but lay around the house, wondering why I hurt."

Up to this point, Chip Tewelk had been in the hospital twice, and in clinics. He'd been treated by three psychiatrists, two neurologists, one oral surgeon, one chiropractor, one physical therapist, and several general practitioners. "My father paid over $250,000 in medical bills," he said. No wonder!"

The irony is that with one or two exceptions, the treatment he received was not misdirected or mistaken—at least, not as far as I could tell, from the medical records I received, but they somehow just missed putting it all together. Some doctors treated the headache, others treated the depression, but nobody seemed to treat the headache and the depression together. They just barely missed doing what the headache specialist would do—go after the pain first, knowing it was a symptom of depression, while trying to relieve the depression itself.

In any event, one of the women in Chip Tewelk's family was browsing through a copy of *Good Housekeeping* magazine one summer day when she came across an article on how specialists in medicine are treating headache patients. She showed it to Chip Tewelk and his father. A number of able specialists were mentioned in that article. I was but one of them, but I was the one that he phoned long distance. He was living in the Southeast and he'd have to visit my office in Chicago.

Chip Tewelk was suffering from chronic posttraumatic headache. I prescribed the MAOI, Nardil. The MAOI worked against the headache and depression at the same time. If the treatment had any dimension other than what he'd experienced before, it was in the assurance that we could keep after the headache pain until it was under control; that we would not offer one treatment and expect that it would work, then quit if it didn't work. In chronic posttraumatic headache, the treatment is geared toward the type headache that is most predominant in the patient's symptoms —if the headache is more

177

migraine-like, then migraine treatment is preferred. If the headache is more tension-type in nature, then treatments one uses for tension-type headache are used.

We did have one other resource and that was the biofeedback technique taught in our office for relieving the pain of the tension features of his headache. For as we've seen, there are biofeedback techniques worked out specifically to help not only migraine but also tension-type headaches. Very conspicuous in all that Chip Tewelk had said, for example, was the feeling of tightening of the muscles in his scalp and neck along with the sensation of pain and pulling on the top of his head. The theory of biofeedback is that the patient can be taught to relax those muscles, and in relaxing them, he will reduce or eliminate the pain.

Chip Tewelk picked up the technique of the biofeedback method readily enough, but he was still rather tentative about it. This, in itself, was a departure from the stereotype. For we expect younger people to be more easily committed to biofeedback than older people. The latter, you would think, would be somewhat more tentative in accepting biofeedback if only because it suggests control of certain body responses—certain human responses—that they were long taught were simply automatic and thus beyond control. The reason that Chip Tewelk, though still in his early 20s, was so tentative about it was because of the abnormal EEG readings he'd had in the past; he felt deep within himself that somehow this would interfere with the "circuitry" involved in the system. Nevertheless, between biofeedback and his medication, he was able to show significant improvement. He was better able to control his tensions and thus his headache pain. It was no miracle cure, but it was encouraging.

Then as it turned out, there was a setback or two. "The headaches in front and top of my head left, although the burning sensation continued, and my neck did not hurt except when lifting," he said. "I began jog, and my neck"— which had been quite rigid, in the manner of the depression victim—"became very loose." Then he was in an automobile accident at home in the spring. He was not seriously injured, but his shoulders and neck began to hurt. In the early

178

summer he was in another accident, and again he was not seriously injured. He said, "basically I was depressed because of the pain and the fear of pain."

He was losing ground now, just at the time he had started building his life back to normal. He had entered summer school, but he was unable to shake a lowering depression. He was coming home, lying on the heating pad, and feeling sorry for himself. But he got control of himself. He applied the principles of relaxation technique of biofeedback and began taking his medicine with more regularity. It was his doing, not mine. I showed him the way and, when threatened with losing his way, he found it again. "The headaches in front and on top stayed away," he said. "The symptoms left, and then the fears left also."

He went back to school in the fall and through to graduation this time. He still had his bad moments. He said, "I went out for life-saving primarily to loosen the muscles in my neck and back. But the idea backfired." He was apprehensive while he was in the pool because he was afraid he'd hurt his neck. "The cervical area was always tight and with poor circulation." That was a continuing fear. "If I go out and play basketball or softball, I tighten my neck and my shoulders. The blood seems not to flow normally in these areas." But he does not let that awareness escalate into a headache.

He had been working on the biofeedback because he wanted to be off drugs. As I've said, he was not totally confident in his ability to use the biofeedback because of the abnormal EEG readings he'd had in the past, but at least he tried. "Since January I've been decreasing my medication," he wrote to me some time later. "I went off it completely but became completely disoriented three or four days later, so I went back on it on a reduced basis."

It was a long hard fight for Chip Tewelk, but he got the headaches under control—"I see myself now as being much better off, being free from the pain of headache. I have come to the point where I can better understand the whole mess."

He still has certain fears and he knows it, but he's better able to cope with them. He is not alone in having fear, nor is he alone in having depression and chronic posttraumatic headache. He had learned to control them.

23

THE MIGRAINE WITHOUT PAIN

He was a structural draftsman, and his eyes were going bad. He was a spry, small-boned man in his 30s. His was a clerical face—mustached, a trifle pinched, with a look of chronic apprehension about it. Every once in a while, he'd experience blurring of his vision—a near blindness in some cases—that would last for 25 to 45 minutes. So far, at work he could take the time to get through it.

"But what would be the consequences if I suffered an attack while driving?" he asked. And what be the consequences if the blurring of vision continued and extended? He might become isolated *in* his job because he could not see the entirety of his work, and he might become isolated *from* it if he couldn't drive along or well enough to get to his office.

He did the natural thing: He went to an eye specialist. The doctor could find nothing wrong with his vision. "In fact, my vision was slightly better than 20-20," he said. But the eye doctor suggested, rather wisely, that he seek out a headache specialist.

When I saw him, I perceived a classic mystery of medicine. There was every reason why he should have migraine, except for the chief one. His mother had migraine. His problems with his vision imitated the first manifestation of migraine—the aura that precedes the pain, but there was no pain.

I prescribed some medication. It didn't work. I tried some other medication and that didn't work. His vision was still blurring. You can see why: in abortive therapy a triptan isn't consumed until the first sign of trouble, and his first signal *was* trouble.

We tried one drug after another until it appeared no antimigraine drug would work. Finally, he made a troubled suggestion to the effect that perhaps it was something of a more "physical" nature. In short, he feared an organic problem. He was amenable to having an MRI, so we scheduled him into the hospital. We gave him a battery of tests and found nothing, except that he was a superbly healthy individual.

Now we were back at the start. I prescribed the beta blocker propranolol for him to take every day to prevent the attacks.

But I was still bothered by the case, and so I went into my library and found some references to a comparable problem by Dr. Walter C. Alvarez, who himself has migraine. He wrote:

"Once when I had a scotoma [the aura before onset of a migraine] as I was driving my car along a narrow country road, I must have had a left hemianopsia [blind spot] because suddenly I discovered a car a few yards away, bearing down on me. I had not seen it as it approached. It is curious that just before this happened, I was not conscious of this decided defect in the left half of my field of vision."

So, Dr. Alvarez had known what my patient suffered and the draftsman clearly had migraine. With that insight, I felt more confident in my diagnosis and the decision to prescribe propranolol. Within a few weeks, the draftsman's attacks became much less frequent and severe. At his last follow-up appointment, he reported to have gone more than one year without a single episode of migraine.

His problem was rare in that it was a migraine without pain, but it was not rare in that it provided a scotoma, or aura, which deeply affected his vision. A good many migraine patients, those who *do* have pain, also suffer these dramatic changes in vision. Not all of them suffer a loss of vision; some of the victims see such extraordinary sights that they feel they are suffering hallucinations.

Most migraine sufferers are threatened with being cut off from a personal sense of achievement, which is a major need in this group of people, and eventually with being cut off from society by the intensity and frequency of their pain. Or, like the patient in this chapter, their work and their privilege of

182

doing what they like best are threatened by their migraine. For although his was a migraine without pain, it had, in cutting of his vision at unpredictable moments, a potentially disastrous impact. Persistence by the headache-oriented physician and the patient will usually solve the most bizarre and catastrophic of migraine mysteries.

24

THE PAIN AFTER SEX

The phone call came at 4 o'clock in the morning. It was a family medicine physician, a friend and associate of mine at the hospital where we are both on the staff. He'd just arranged to have a patient of his, 32-year-old Stanley Alwed, admitted to the hospital as an emergency patient.

"The symptom," he said, "is a very intense and uncontrollable headache. The pain is focused behind both of his eyes. He experienced sudden and severe vomiting."

"Did the headache wake him out of a sound sleep?" You remember that cluster headache, which strikes suddenly and involves very intense pain, seems to come on, for the first time, in the dead of night and awaken the victim out of a sound sleep. "No, he was awake. He'd just completed sexual intercourse, had an orgasm, and then the headache struck him."

This physician was alert. There are, perhaps, some physicians who would have dismissed the fact that the headache pain came on after intercourse as being incidental or unimportant. My colleague recognized it as being quite significant.

"One more thing," said the doctor. "He has a very stiff neck."

That was not irrelevant. It was a most important piece of information. In fact, it was all coming together, in a thoroughly ominous way.

"I think," I said, "I'd better get down to the hospital right away."

At the hospital, the patient told us of the searing headache pain. It seemed to start in the front of his head and radiate all the way to the back. The pain was so great, and the vomiting so sudden and violent, that he felt impelled to wake up his doctor in the middle of the night. And his doctor responded with precisely the proper emergency care. Later in the morning, when the patient was

185

more relaxed, we gave him the needed neurological exams. The MRI did not suggest any organic problems.

But he still did have a very stiff neck and usually this is indicative of something serious. As you may recall, victims of tension-type headaches, often have a stiff neck. The stiffness of neck was clearly due to some other problem. There were a half-dozen, perhaps even more, possibilities. To accumulate the clues and to narrow the possibilities down to one certainty, I ordered several further examinations.

In a spinal tap, the physician inserts a needle into the spinal column and removes a small amount of fluid from it. This is the fluid that surrounds the brain and the spinal column and cushions them both from shock. It usually flows from the brain area down into the spinal column that out of the brain cavity, and from it we get certain clues as to what's happening organically in or around the brain.

One thing to be aware of in performing a spinal tap is that too much fluid might easily be withdrawn during the puncture. If too much fluid is drawn out and thus lost to the cerebrospinal system, the brain loses some of its cushion fluid and drops down slightly lower in the skull. When the brain does drop, it pulls on the arteries and other matter in its supportive structure, and that pulling causes pain—a headache. It usually takes several days for the body to regenerate enough fluid to rebuild the cushion around and under the brain. The headache will continue all through that time, until the cushion is built up again. So under the best of conditions, the spinal tap must be performed with care and with accuracy.

In this case, we had a specific reason for performing the spinal tap. The stiff neck is often an indication that a patient has some kind of foreign or irritating factor in the spinal fluid. It was all the more likely since the neurological examinations gave us certain indications of what was *not* happening in the patient's skull.

What we found in the spinal fluid of Stanley Alwed was a surprising amount of blood. There are several reasons why blood might turn up in significant quantities in the spinal fluid. One is, obviously, a hemorrhage of the blood vessels in or around the brain. If a massive breakage has occurred, the patient will often get a severe headache and then—as the blood flows out through the break in the blood vessel—he'll become unconscious and often he will die. (President Franklin Roosevelt died of a massive cerebral hemorrhage. His last words were, before he slumped into unconsciousness, "I have a terrific headache.")

There are, of course, lesser hemorrhages that also include headaches. They involve not major blood vessels but small capillaries. They do not involve the whole head but only a small portion of the brain. But when the blood spills out, there is no immediate fresh supply of blood to that portion of the brain, and blood carries the oxygen which the brain needs for life. So without blood, the brain is without oxygen, and without oxygen the cells in the bloodless portion of the brain die. Their death causes anything from a small speech difficulty or a drooping eyelid to a major paralysis. It is possible for modern medicine to treat these "strokes" so that the patient has a chance to make a partial or complete recovery.

But a hemorrhage is not the only reason that blood will turn up in the spinal fluid. Sometimes it is produced from a leakage though what are called angiomas. They are enlarged blood vessels, and they can appear anywhere, on the skin, for example, as well as in the brain. (One version of them, often found on the face and made up of bright or purple-red capillaries, is commonly called Mother's Mark.) When in the brain they do not need to rupture to produce blood in the spinal column; they are capable of leaking just a very little blood which will turn up in the spinal fluid.

Still another possibility is an aneurysm. This is a bulging out of a blood vessel, something like a small blown-up balloon, appearing suddenly in the brain. It happens in a weak spot in the wall of a blood vessel. You imagine it

187

best by picturing a weak spot in an inner tube; it bulges out and, as it does so, the wall of the bulge gets thinner and thinner until there's a "blowout." That's the danger of the aneurysm: it may blow out before you notice it. And the blowout, because it's large, usually leads to such massive hemorrhaging of blood that death is inevitable—and virtually immediate.

But there is also a chance that blood will seep through the thinned-out walls of the aneurysm before they rupture. The aneurysm "weeps" blood, so to speak, and that blood sinks down through the fluid cushion of the brain into the fluid in the spinal column. By measuring the amount of blood in the spinal fluid that's withdrawn through the spinal tap, you get an idea of whether you've got an aneurysm "weeping" in the brain or a tiny capillary that is hemorrhaging. (If it's a huge hemorrhage, you won't need to measure the blood in the spinal fluid to find out about it.)

To narrow these possibilities down further, we asked Stanley Alwed to undergo yet another examination, an MRA (magnetic resonance angiogram).

In this case, the angiogram showed clearly a gathering of dye and blood—because the dye was still being carried in the blood—in a bulge in a particular part of one of the arteries of the brain. It was not characteristic of a brain tumor or a blood clot, and it did not show any leaking or "weeping," but it was characteristic of an aneurysm.

As you might guess, this is a most serious condition. For you never quite know when the "balloon" will burst. And yet you must do nothing when the aneurysm is "hot," as this man's was, for it is very sensitive. Its extreme sensitivity causes the pain, and it became sensitive because of the unusual stress on the cardiovascular system with sexual intercourse. Women as well as men will be attacked by the pain of an aneurysm, if they have one, during, or after intercourse. This patient had, in fact, been attacked by such headaches on earlier occasions, though never by headaches of this intensity. (Either sex will also be attacked by the pain of aneurysm when they engage in any extreme exertion that

188

will put undue pressure on the cardiovascular system, such as lifting heavy weights for extended periods of time.)

One thing to note about headaches such as these is that they are vascular headaches; that is to say, they involve the swelling of a blood vessel. It happens that it is one blood vessel and that is extremely swollen, but the principle is the same.

In fact, an aneurysm seems to mimic migraine, the best known of the vascular headaches. Some doctors will diagnose an aneurysm headache as migraine. The headache does appear first in the forehead, behind one or both eyes, and it involves a very intense, regular throbbing pain. But the point of a medical examination is to explore the subtleties of the patient's complaints—and the improbabilities of it.

Not long ago, for example, we had a woman come into our Headache Clinic who complained of a fierce and sudden onset of migraine. It attacked on one side of the head. It lasted for hours, then went away, and came back later. There was only one mystifying factor: she was 65 years old, and migraine very rarely attacks a woman of that age for the first time. The doctor has to ask himself why it would suddenly turn up in this one woman at this singular age. If he asks himself this question, and if he knows that migraines usually pass, not start, after menopause, then he is going to seek other reasons for the headache pain. She had an aneurysm that was hot. We gave it time to cool down and then took a good close look at it through an angiogram. It promised trouble. For it was in a part of the brain that could not be reached through surgery.

We couldn't do anything about it. It would just have to stay there, a living time bomb in her head. To be sure, we could treat her, and it, with medication. There's always the chance that it might be cooled and perhaps reduced. But nobody knows when suddenly it might swell up like an old rubber inner tube and blow out. It could happen tomorrow; it might not happen for 10 years.

In the case of Stanley Alwed, there was happier news. His aneurysm was in an accessible part of the brain. We just kept him in bed with complete and uncompromising rest for 14 days. The idea was to give the aneurysm a chance to cool down. Without any strain on his part, aside from breathing regularly, we felt we could reduce the inflammation of the side walls of the bulge. In fact, a lot of people who don't know they have aneurysms unconsciously take the same therapy when it's forced on them by the headache of the aneurysm: they stop and lie down and relax until the pain goes away. In that time, the aneurysm starts to cool down. It doesn't get cured. Its danger of rupture is simply allayed for a while, how short a while, nobody knows.

But in the hospital, we were able to treat the patient with medication which would help cool down the aneurysm. The idea was to prepare him for surgery. When he was ready, the surgeon simply went into his skull at the point of the aneurysm. The idea is to ligate, or tie off the blood vessel at the base of the aneurysm. You'll hear doctors talk about "going in and putting a clip on it." The "clip" is the system for tying off the artery. In that way, the blood will be redirected in to the balance of the healthy artery when, and if, the aneurysm blows out. The reason: the entrance to the ballooning portion of the blood vessel is tied off, with a clip, before the blowout occurs. Thus the balloon may deflate because blood is no longer flowing through it. And the blood is redirected so that no brain cells die off from a lack of oxygen.

In the case of Stanley Alwed, the ligation was made smoothly and simply. He was in the hospital for another five days. His recovery was complete and successful.

25

THE BOY WITH THE BRAIN TUMOR

He was a compelling child with dark, liquid eyes and small for his age. He was 14, and he looked like a 9-year-old. He was a bright boy, very conscientious about his schoolwork, very aware of his grades, which were good. His father was a janitor, his parents loved him and were proud of him, and gave him something cherished in this world that many other children miss and never know they miss, love. In the end, he was a youngster who could face tragedy and pain.

He came to us one bright summer afternoon on the recommendation of his family doctor, with a pain all over his head. The pain was constant; it had started the previous October and had not quit since then. But sometimes, perhaps three or four times a week, it would reach a peak and then recede. He had difficulty falling asleep. He tended to wake up early in the morning with the headache already going.

Chronic migraine? Possibly, when you consider that migraine does attack children even younger than this boy. Before puberty, little boys have migraine as often as little girls. Moreover, he had blurred vision and nausea, and he did vomit quite a bit. He had an uncle with migraine, and he exhibited some of the personality of a migraine patient. He had ambition and goals, and he was a perfectionist.

And so, our first tentative diagnosis was for chronic migraine. But there were things that bothered me in describing his pain as a migraine. There was something wrong about those other symptoms: the boy had blurred vision and nausea and vomiting but not necessarily in association with the headache pain. He would not have them just before the pain started reaching for its peak as in migraine. Instead these other symptoms might come on at any time. Another primary symptom was pain on exertion, and if you have an increase of pain or the onset of pain with exertion, one should always look for an organic cause, such as a brain tumor.

The medical history that his father sent along to me showed that the boy had been under care of a "nervous stomach," and that he had allergies to dust, pollens, molds, and some animals. This could explain some of the stomach unrest, and perhaps the allergies could explain the headache pain. But why didn't the headache pain come on him earlier? Why had it come on so recently and so suddenly?

I kept thinking migraine but suspecting something else. We gave the youngster a neurological exam, but there was no sign of trouble. We then scheduled an MRI (Magnetic Resonance Imaging). MRI uses a strong magnetic field and radio waves to create detailed images of the organs and tissues within the body. The MRI revealed a brain tumor. The tumor was located in the cerebellum, the lower or back part of the brain that has to do with motor coordination and equilibrium, which would help explain why he had vertigo. However, this is an area that is difficult to reach through brain surgery.

One day in the hospital, this boy, so full of charm and appeal, just looked at me in the eye and asked, "Do I have a brain tumor?"

This is the ultimate question facing any doctor. For it intimates, "Am I going to die?" It was one which I'd faced with my own father. He had terminal cancer, and it was apparent to him that something was gravely wrong. The question was whether and how to tell him. I've always taken the position that we should wait until the patient asks. If the patient wants to know, he'll ask, and I'll give that patient a direct, honest answer. But if a patient doesn't ask, I don't force it on him.

My father never asked. But he was a wise enough man, who knew enough about medicine, to understand much of what I didn't tell him. It was just that he was not the kind who would ask. (Needless to say, it is important to tell the immediate family of the patient, and they may tell the patient. For it may be important to have a will made out or brought up to date, and the patient's cooperation is necessary for that. In such a case, the doctor may find himself confirming the worst by confirming the need for a will.)

When my f14-year-old patient asked, I felt compelled to tell him the truth.

"Yes, you have a brain tumor," I told him. "But I think we can cure it."

It took an operation consuming almost six hours. In the opening phase of the operation, the surgeon and those of us attending him could see what had caused the headaches. The tumor had blocked the normal flow of fluid from the brain down into the spine. It was building up pressure in the cranium and the pressure was causing the headache. So, the operation demanded first a shunt, the installation of a little plastic tube that would carry the fluid around the tumor so that the flow was not interrupted. That relieved the pressure within the brain.

As the operation continued, it became clear that the surgeon, however skilled, would not be able to get all of the tumor even though he was using a new innovation called the Gamma Knife. Gamma Knife is not actually a knife at all, but a device that concentrates cobalt radiation into a small space for the treatment of brain tumors. It was invented at the Karolinska Institute in Sweden. The samples sent to pathology indicated positively that it was malignant. But there was one alternative: this type of tumor was quite susceptible to radiation.

So, the operation was concluded and, after the boy recovered from surgery, cobalt radiation was begun. It seemed to be successful. In the period following radiation, there appeared to be no impact from the remnant of the tumor. Except from the boy himself. He'd been fitted out with a wig after surgery because his head had been shaved. He'd also been given private tutoring to keep up with his schooling. He liked both. In fact, he wouldn't give up the wig or the tutoring until his hair had fully grown back. And I got the very strong impression that he was going to be the ultimate judge of that.

In any event, we cured his headache, which was a small enough achievement. We found the cause of the headache and medicine—through surgery and radiation—managed to cure it.

Will the cure hold?

We hope so. There is, in such cases, the legendary five-year-period: if the patient survives without a renewal of the problem, then it is considered cured. In cases where the patient has this kind of tumor, a medulloblastoma of the cerebellum, there might be suggestions of further caution. Some patients have been known to succumb 20 or 25 years later.

But we shared the gift of life with this boy, and that was a reward in itself.

26

THE EX-INFANTRYMAN

It is a myth. It is not true that headache victims are somehow, in ways subtle or obvious, weaker than the rest of us. It is not true that they collapse under stress. It is simply that they are attacked by a particular kind of pain for reasons which they themselves cannot altogether recognize.

About 20 years ago, Gregory Wilson was a squarely built, chesty man of 50 who wore his authority with easy assurance. His black, bushy hair was edged with gray. He talked in short, staccato phrases. His father was one of the most famous men in journalism and he himself had built a formidable career in business: he was one of the top public relations men in one of the largest corporations in the United States. He was a hard-driving man who liked to busy himself outside of his job with other writing projects. He was as successful in them as he was in the rest of his career.

Some 16 years ago he had been attacked by severe and recurring headaches. There is every indication that he had a migraine personality and he, for one, was convinced that they were migraine. He remained convinced of that, although I disagreed with him.

Although he was in a stress-filled job, he was not easy prey to stress of an exceptional kind.

He had been a combat infantryman during two tours in Vietnam, and he suffered no particular stress under the most violent conditions. He did not even suffer from lack of sleep. Early in the 1990s, he took a year's leave of absence from work to run for Congress. It did nothing but make him feel better.

"Despite a grueling 16-hour-day, 7-day-a-week schedule of campaigning which taxed mind and body, I never had a single headache, upset stomach, or sleepless night," he said. "The increased work load and responsibility made me peppier than ever before in my life."

He was in his early 30s when the headaches first became burdensome. He checked with his company physician, underwent a detailed checkup, and found that he was a diabetic. That was strange in terms of migraine action. Diabetics are likely to find that their migraine is reduced, not increased, with the onset of the disease. "I believe your headaches are due to tension," the doctor reported to him. But once the belief was stated, the relief did not follow.

Over the years, he consulted a good many distinguished physicians in New York, Chicago, and elsewhere to seek help for his headaches, but none was forthcoming. One winter he was vacationing in Tucson, Arizona, where he went to an excellent physician for both headaches and diabetes. The doctor gave him a long technical article on headaches to read and he found my name mentioned. He found it again when he returned home and read a story on headaches by a science writer. He knew the writer involved, so he checked me out, and then arranged for an appointment.

We gave him the in-office physical. He'd just had a very extensive battery of hospital tests. Fearful of a brain tumor, he'd checked into one the finest hospitals in Chicago and come out with a report that he was free of tumor or other abnormalities in the brain and skull. But he still had his headaches.

Between the hospital reports and my in-office procedures, we were able to eliminate organic problems as a cause of his headaches. (As for his diabetes, he was taking a bedtime dose of injectable long-acting glargine [Lantus], and he reported that his sugars were well-controlled.)

He was convinced that he had migraine. That was understandable, but I began to look elsewhere, for his headaches were not focused on one side or the other. They came daily, not occasionally. He was troubled by sleep disturbances—he customarily awakened early in the morning. All these were signs of a deep depression that was exhibiting itself in a persistent and intense headache.

Actually, I felt he had chronic migraine. For though the depression was prominent, some of the headaches he suffered, on occasion, to me sounded very

196

much as if they were migraine. So I chose the MAOI—Nardil. I had two reasons for choosing Nardil: It is one of those rare medications which seem to work against depression as well as against migraine; and I did not want to use the common antidepressants, amitriptyline (Elavil), for example, because I felt it might cause complications with his diabetes.

It turned out that the choice was a good one. His headaches were greatly reduced right from the start. As time went by, he seemed to overcome them altogether. He saw other benefits from the medication. "I no longer lose my temper over sloppy work and my patience quota has risen sharply," he said.

But the second phase of treatment failed somewhat. I was, of course, curious professionally and personally at what might be causing the depression. For here was a man who had endured combat and politics without any headache problems or sleep disturbance. And suddenly in his 30s and 40s he fell prey to both.

I thought it might have to do with his married life. There were indications that he was not getting on well with his wife and some of the headache patterns—their increase during vacations and weekends—suggested an effort to maintain calm in a situation which he found difficult. But when I asked him about it, he was quite blunt. He didn't want to talk about it. He told me he didn't consult me as a psychiatrist. Thus the barriers were high and formidable. When somebody tells me that, I leave him alone.

We'd conquered the pain, and that was his top concern. He was aware, I'm sure, of the conflict that brought about depression. And he was learning to live with it or to live apart from it: he separated from his wife. He was not a weak man; his whole life showed that, and once he was freed from pain, he was also free to tackle, by himself, the problem behind it.

In subsequent years, whenever my name appeared in relation to headache he would send me a note and a copy of the article and tell me in his note how well he was doing. He died recently of other causes than his headache but donated a very substantial amount of his fortune to the National Headache

Foundation.

27

THE COMPULSIVE DRUG-TAKER

At home, one Sunday morning in the spring, I received an urgent phone call from a woman who had to see me, she insisted, right away. It was more than a matter of pain; it was a matter of the survival of her marriage. And so I agreed to an immediate appointment.

In a way, I was startled when we met. She was a woman approaching 60. She had a drawn face and a distraught manner. She had migraine, which is in itself somewhat unusual. For in the vast majority of cases, the pain of migraine declines or disappears after a woman has gone through menopause, or middle age, because of the lower production of female hormones in her body.

I was startled also because a first step in quelling or controlling those headaches turned up in our first few minutes of conversation. It developed that she had been taking hormone tablets for years, partly out of fear she would lose her femininity after menopause. Those pills, I was sure, were contributing to or causing her migraine. By asking her to give up the hormones, I was sure that I could reduce the intensity and frequency of her pain. And, as it turned out, I was right. As it turned out, also, that was not her ultimate problem.

"My husband is about to leave me," she said. Her lips trembled and the words came out all in a rush, and not with a great degree of comprehension. When I sorted it all through, her husband, whom she still loved deeply, had warned her that she had to do something about her headaches. But that was a code word, or a code system. What he was really warning her was that she had to do something about her pill-popping.

For this woman had become habituated to her medicine, Norco, which contains the opioid hydrocodone together with acetaminophen. There are withdrawal symptoms from sudden stoppage of opioids. This woman was, for example, taking 14 pills a day; that's almost 100 tablets a week.

199

So she was in a terrible cycle. She was taking hormones which were increasing her headaches, she was taking Norco to help reduce the pain of her headaches, and she was convinced that she needed both—the Norco perhaps more than the hormones. For if she went off the hormones, she might still feel a need to take the Norco.

"You simply have to help me get off these drugs," she said, "or my husband will leave me."

The question of drug dependence is one which must always arise in medicine, as the concern of doctors as well as patients. You simply cannot practice medicine and work in the field of pain without knowing of the danger of drug dependence, or drug habituation. The most urgent imperative is that the doctor not habituate a patient deliberately in an effort to overcome the patient's pain. The next most urgent imperative is that the doctor not even let it happen casually. In this patient's case, her primary care physician prescribed her Norco and continued to refill it without many questions, and often he did not see her in his office for more than six months at a time. In reality, he enabled her to become—and to continue to be—addicted to Norco.

We try to avoid this in our office by keeping very close track of the nature and impact—the habituating effects as well as side effects—of the drugs we prescribe. In the case of opioids, we do not refill the medication without seeing the patient at the very least every three months. In fact, opioids have a very limited utility in the treatment of migraine. If opioids are to be a part of the treatment regimen, their use should be limited to no more than 8-10 days per month. Exceeding that limit puts the patient not only at greater risk of dependence, but it also sets the stage for the development of medication overuse headache (MOH).

Now, of course, patients who do become dependent on a drug have many strategies for building up a supply of that drug. They will phone the office and say, "Oh, I just knocked a brand-new bottle of that drug in the toilet. Could you be a sweet thing and call the pharmacist for a refill for me?" Or they'll call long distance when they're on a trip and say, "Oh, I forgot my medicine in the rush to leave. Would you be a dear and call up a pharmacist here and have him fill it for me so I don't come down with the headaches while I'm on this trip." Of course, these things can actually happen to nondrug-dependent persons. So in my office, I have a system for keeping track of such requests from our patients. If they are repeated over and over again, we spot it as a warning that the patient is becoming drug dependent, or became drug dependent before he or she came to see me.

Some of those in the pain field, including those specializing in the treatment of headaches, lay down a simple law: "Never use an addictive drug on a patient with pain." It is, in fact, very difficult to avoid using the most powerful and addictive painkillers under certain circumstances. We don't have occasion to use morphine in the treatment of headache, but it is not difficult to imagine other doctors in the field of pain using it in very severe or emergency cases (perhaps in terminal cancer when the patient is near death). It is simply given only where the conditions are such that the patient will not suffer an enduring dependence. Even in the field of headache pain, I occasionally use very powerful drugs—methadone, for example—to help a patient in extreme pain. But this is not done casually; it is done only with complete knowledge of the drug's impact, with repeated warnings to the patient, and with safeguards in our office so that a drug dependence does not develop.

To be sure, a good many of the drug-dependent cases that we see involve a dependence built up through earlier treatment, perhaps by nonspecialists. The most conscientious physicians not in constant contact with certain drugs in the pain field find it hard to be aware of the subtleties of many drugs. To a large extent, this is the fault of the pharmaceutical manufacturers who fail to warn doctors adequately of the dangers of drug dependency with some of their concoctions.

There are several drugs which tend to get their victims dependent or habituated. They all pose an additional problem for the doctor who treats these patients. For the physician must attack the problem of drug dependency before he or she can attack the problem of headache pain. There are very eminent doctors in the field of headache pain who simply will not treat a patient who is drug dependent. "Go break the habit, then come back and see me," they say. It is very difficult for the patients to do so because in the pain of headache they have the motive for taking the drug, as well as the very powerful desire to take it. The truth is, you see some very impressive men and women come into your office and find they're dependent on their drugs.

One time the father of one of my students in the medical school where I teach came in to see me with a migraine problem. He was an executive of a major steel firm and the headaches were, of course, interfering with his work. His problem was more than migraine: he had developed a dependence on Percocet (which is oxycodone, an opioid, together with acetaminophen), which had been prescribed earlier by another doctor. Also in this case, the physician continued to refill the Percocet with little or no question and rarely seeing the patient. The son, realizing what was going on and perceiving what it was doing to his father, urged him to come see me.

I laid it out for him: he had to be willing to break with the drug. I'd help him do it. I'd help treat the pain of his migraine. I'd help him get the migraine headaches under control, but he had to level with me. He'd have to give up his drug (see Appendix II for a discussion on inpatient therapy for drug dependence).

Of course, he said he would, and of course, he didn't mean it. Perhaps the discipline was too hard, even for a successful businessman. For he was trying to solve both the drug dependence and the headache pain and they are very difficult problems to tackle. You can appreciate how a patient might feel that if he or she keeps one problem (the drug dependence), he or she can attack the other problem (that of the headache pain), and that's a lot easier than trying to tackle both problems at once.

In any case, this patient simply drifted off when it became clear to both of us that he wasn't going to shake his drug dependence. My guess is that he's simply going to live out his life depending on the drug whether or not the headaches stay with him.

Another case involved a man with an enormously attractive personality, a man with sculpted gray-white hair and strong features, who was then approaching the age of 50. He was a Roman Catholic priest, and he was stationed at a well-known, though small, non-secular college; I could well imagine that he was a favorite of the students, Catholic and non-Catholic, at that college. Some years earlier, he'd been treated by somebody else for migraine without aura. In the course of the treatment, he'd been given a prescription for Nubain, which is another opioid. He was to take it by injection. It must have made him feel somewhat better, for he started taking it twice a week, then three times a week, then four times a week. By the time I saw him, he was completely hooked. He was taking it in three injections a day, but he was combining several ampules in each injection. So he was taking 60-80 milligrams a day of this very potent drug.

He realized he had a problem, but he had no organized way of attacking it. He rationalized that it was the headaches and not the drug that prompted him to take so much of the Nubain. In fact, he had a psychological and physical dependence on the drug (as in heroin addiction, where there is also a physical as well as psychological need for the drug). So he sought a nondrug method of attacking the headache pain.

It was a very logical decision, and it led him into an exploration of biofeedback as a nondrug treatment for migraine. He read about biofeedback and he went to Topeka, Kansas, and the Menninger Clinic, the home, so to speak, of biofeedback treatment of migraine.

Today I wish I could say we had an unqualified success. But I simply don't know. The patient comes in every three to six months. He seems better, in terms of his headache. He says the biofeedback helped, and I'm sure the

203

sumatriptan I prescribed helped, but I'm never quite sure. I keep feeling that somewhere, somehow, the good father is getting a large daily dose of Nubain. I don't prescribe it for him, but I have that very definite, very profound feeling that for a man with his personality it is not altogether impossible to get as much as he needs through irregular sources. The only thing that can truly be said is that if he's kidding me, he's also kidding himself.

There is still another case that came to my office that involved an escalating and even weird kind of tragedy. The patient was a very well-to-do man who'd suffered migraine attacks since he was five or six years old. But the migraine was of a very special kind: It was abdominal migraine. That is to say, he had the visual aura and later he had nausea and vomiting. But he didn't get migraine pains in the head: he got them in his abdomen. This is rare but not unknown; abdominal migraine is a symptom which appears and reappears all through the medical literature on migraine pain.

The difficulty is that not an awful lot of primary care providers were or are reading the literature on migraine pain. And so when they encountered this child who had intense pains—incredibly intense pains with a dull, constant throbbing—in the abdomen, they felt that he suffered a very severe disease of the abdomen. That's quite natural. Right?

In this case, they figured on everything from ulcers to cancer. To find out, they did the simple and direct thing: They cut him open to take a look at his abdomen. They didn't find anything, so they closed him up, until the next series of abdominal migraine pains. Then they opened him up again and took another look. They didn't find anything, so they closed him up again. Altogether, this man had major surgery on his abdomen five times while he was a young boy. Of course they didn't find anything, for migraine pain doesn't leave any organic signs.

But as so often happens, the abdominal migraine eventually moved to the head and became the kind of migraine-of-the-head that we all might recognize. That did not make it much easier on him, it just made it easier on the doctors. For he went through a number of them, and although they couldn't get rid of his headaches, they at least recognized the cause of the pain.

When I finally saw him, he was a tall, thin man in his middle 40s. He was a manufacturer and he was both successful and rich. He'd been referred to me by another doctor who treated him for the migraine, and somehow left him hooked on Oxycontin (oxycodone). Perhaps because he had enough money, he always found a way to get as much of it as he needed.

This particular patient was taking excessive amounts of Oxycontin twice a day. He had the problem of addiction in addition to migraine, and the addiction demanded treatment as well. I recommended that he be admitted to our inpatient headache unit. We sought the assistance of an addiction medicine physician during his hospital stay. Although he did go through withdrawal symptoms from the opioids during the hospital stay, he was able to be discharged after 10 days and reported his headache had improved significantly. At his first follow-up one month later, however, he had returned to taking opioids prescribed by another physician.

I think we did something for his headaches. I'm not sure we did anything for his addiction. But the situation became moot because he became involved in certain marital difficulties that made it hard for me to treat him further.

All of this by way of explanation and background for the case of the women who phoned me on Sunday morning in the spring. The story emphasizes how serious is the matter of drug dependency.

The best way to wean people off drugs of this kind is simply to put them under very controlled conditions for a certain length of time. Thus, I recommended that she enter the hospital. She spent $2^1/_2$ weeks there. During that time, I managed to get her off the hormones which were contributing to her migraine pain. More important, I helped her break her dependency on Norco. The migraine pain came under control, the drug dependency disappeared, and I sent her home, perhaps cured, certainly drug-free.

Eight months passed. I would see her occasionally, principally to monitor how her migraine control was going. It was very effective, thanks to the fact that she was free of hormones. It became an incidental matter to talk about her one-time drug dependency, for it no longer preoccupied her.

Then, on another Sunday morning, this time in the winter, she phoned again, and again she was desperate. She'd gone back on the Talwin three or four weeks earlier. There'd been a family crisis with one of her children and she'd retreated to pill-popping—to drug dependency—as solace in that crisis. Now she was afraid she was hooked again. And she was faced with that further crisis: Her husband knew, and he was renewing his decision to leave. Her request was simple: "Will you please hospitalize me and get me off these pills again?"

I did. She was in the hospital this time for just over a week, and again she broke her drug dependency. She showed no signs of the intense migraine pain. The migraine was very infrequent and very low level when it struck at all.

She went home again drug-free. By and large, she continued at home pain-free. I didn't even have to give her any medication for the migraine. Just staying off the hormones seemed to work.

The important thing is that she had the courage to break the dependency. To be sure, she had the motive: The fear of losing her husband whom she loved. But given that motive, she found a way to break the habit as well as to curb the migraine.

28

THE MANIPULATED TRAGEDY

In studying these pages, you may have detected a certain beat, an indefinable momentum. It is simply that everything, in the final analysis, seems to work— pain is muted, tragedy is overcome, justice and virtue are rewarded. Well, this *is* the way it happens most of the time. But there is a side to reality that is shadowed. Sometimes things don't work; sometimes the tragedy is heightened; sometimes justice and virtue are forgotten in the scramble for simple survival.

This is the story about one such case. I'm not sure where the failure lay, whether it was with me or with the patient or with such tempestuous forces of personality that all the power of medicine could not control them. But certainly matters did not come to a successful conclusion; in fact, they came to a tragic end.

The patient was a woman of middle years. She was a dramatics teacher, one who had been quite successful at her career in her early years. She was married to a high school principal. For a long while they lived in a small-to middle-sized eastern community where she performed her work with skill and satisfaction and where her husband had a large school and a very responsive student body. At the time, she had migraine. It was migraine with aura and it had bothered her, though only occasionally, ever since her teens. Then about seven or eight years before I met her, the headaches became more severe and more frequent. Soon they were appearing two or three times weekly; indeed, they were so frequent and intense that they began interfering with her work.

Why did the headaches increase so severely at that time? We can only reconstruct today what happened then. It is possible that she began taking hormones to offset the impact of menopause. Or it is just as possible that she began developing a very difficult and stress-filled environment for herself. For one thing, she had her work; that was demanding in itself. For another thing, she had her family and her duties to it, and then she had a special role as wife of the principal who had the biggest school in the entire area. Thus she had a social as well as professional role.

On a different level of speculation, we might consider what impact the headaches were having on those around her. There was a suggestion later that she used the headaches to manipulate her family—to get them to do precisely what she wanted when she wanted it. If they hesitated, if they had second thoughts, if they simply sought a different or better way to do things, she would suddenly come down with a terrible pain in her head.

Thus, pain became in her hands and head a powerful weapon. There are headache victims who know how to use their pain. They simply manipulate people in every direction in order to get their own way. There is a very good chance that they do not genuinely want to give up their pain. Without it, they cannot control their environment. So although they may seem to seek relief from their headache pain, they do not really want to give it up. The pain is very, very valuable to them—when it is used in a ruthless way.

That is one of the reasons why we counsel the nurses in our office and hospital not to be overly sympathetic to patients who come in continually displaying their pain. Our nurses are taught not only to be professionally and personally efficient, but to be happy and positive and help build an environment which is cheerful and forward-looking rather than dolorous and turned inward. The nurses are much more inclined to exult with a patient who is overcoming pain than to sit down and tut-tut endlessly with a patient who is forever displaying pain as a personal cross to bear. They have the feeling, as I do, that the patients are going to get well and that we're all going to work toward that goal.

In this particular case, there is evidence that the patient used her pain in such a way as to compromise her husband's professional position; that may have been reflexive. I was to feel, later, that she believed she'd made an unsuitable or unhappy marriage. There are, of course, some women and men who inevitably set out to destroy their spouse or their marriages. They do not divorce their spouse, but simply murder them by small degrees. I cannot explore today what was happening within the family at that time. But there did seem to be degeneration within the family. The children moved away, their father was later to tell me that they could not tolerate the discipline-by-pain that their mother imposed. They suffered from her headaches as much as she did, perhaps more, and so did their father. For it seems that his performance as a principal was not altogether successful. I do not know why, but he had transferred from his school to another, a small, school in the far West. There may have been a feeling within the family that the headaches of the wife were at least partly implicated.

When she came to me, I found that she'd been treated, more than adequately, I might add, by a neurologist in her former hometown. The only notable thing is that she was taking an unusual amount of codeine and Fiorinal. I tried to wean her off of them and turn instead to preventive medication, because codeine is somewhat too powerful and often habit-forming. Usually, anybody habituated cannot be treated on an outpatient basis; it is best to admit them to an inpatient headache unit. The significant thing in this case is that, as I insisted more and more she give up earlier drugs, the headaches got worse and worse. The prophylactic medicines didn't seem to have any effect.

I tried other combinations, and I put a no-refill order on the codeine and Fiorinal. The idea was to prevent the headaches from getting started, not to try to kill the pain with codeine after it got a big head start. Then our office began noting a pattern. The patient phoned to say that she'd just accidentally knocked her codeine into the toilet and asked me to write a new prescription. Or she was off visiting old friends in her former home and she'd forgotten the codeine. Could my office tell the local pharmacist? All the familiar devices. I decided to clamp down harder on her intake of codeine.

That elicited a letter from her. Its burden was that life is difficult enough for a person who doesn't respond favorably to treatment, particularly to the preventive system of medication, without having the simpler remedies taken away from her. Her pain was, after all, too great to ignore.

And then suddenly I realized: Hey! She's trying to manipulate me with her pain just as she'd been manipulating her husband and children. If I tried to take her codeine away from her, she'd make sure her headaches got worse, and she'd let me know that none of my other medication was working so that she had every right to her codeine.

This raised a different and difficult problem. I resolved to try to solve it. That, after all, is the point of my practice—to tackle and solve the most difficult headache problems. Yet the atmosphere was not altogether amiable. Once she commented that she understood that "it would be a lot more rewarding to take care of patients who get well." She was telling me that I was impatient because her headache pain was particularly difficult to conquer. She knew that before she'd come to me and *she* was right all along. Moreover, she didn't much care for the attitude of my nurses. "Your confident young nurses ought to be asked to treat patients as though, in spite of all their magic, they may not get well," she said. She was telling me, and them, that she was a tougher case than they'd ever encountered before. The implicit suggestion was that unless we all shaped up, we'd find out how *really* difficult her case was.

If I thought I had problems, I heard from her husband that I was not alone. Before she'd come in for one of her regular appointments, he'd phone to relate what had been happening at home. When the children came back to visit, they didn't want to stay or even be seen at their family home; they'd go to a friend's house and ask their father to go there to talk to them. They couldn't take the discipline-by-pain routine, even for a while. For his part, things were going slowly in his new position. His wife wanted to redo the house according to her own ideas, and she'd get started on them, but somehow she'd never quite get finished. Of course she *was* busy. She did have migraine with aura, you'll recall, and she had some of the drives of the migraine personality. She decided to begin teaching dramatics again. As a matter of fact, she tried and stopped four times.

210

Something always seemed to get in her way; maybe it was the headaches, maybe it was the codeine.

Meanwhile in the office I as fighting my own little battle. I tried to persuade her that if she'd give up her hormones, there might be a significant decline in, or disappearance of, her headaches. I explained that there was very likely to be a decline in migraine pain after menopause—as long as the migraine-inclined person did not take hormones. Her response was that she knew a woman of 81 who still had headaches and certainly *she* was past menopause.

I pointed out that codeine, in the form that she was taking, might create a dependency. I figured I was being conservative. She figured I was being a wild-eyed radical. She'd been to a lot of other doctors, and they assured her there was no sensitivity to codeine. "So what's all the fuss about? Do I detect a little alarm on your part because I'm trying to lessen the pain?"

I indicated that it wasn't just the codeine, but I felt that perhaps she was overusing triptans. The suggestion was that she might have an inclination to drug dependency which we both should watch out for. So she came back with something along the lines of: "If I act desperate, I am. I wake up every morning with a headache. You don't know how that feels, doctor. To wake up every day with pain. And to have pain all day. It takes codeine and two or three suppositories just to get started. Yesterday, today, every day. There is no exception, doctor. Today is no exception." And then the sweet come-on: "Of course I *have* improved and should continue treatment, but not if we've reached the point where you don't trust me."

Beautiful! Great manipulation! Unless I changed my attitude, and began to appreciate how truly terrible was her pain, she'd have to drop me!

At home, from what her husband told me in his pre-appointment phone calls, things were not really going well. He felt a need to entertain some of his students and teachers in his home as previous principals had done. But now a year had passed and still the home wasn't ready. And he felt he had to apologize

211

all the time to his staff and to his superintendent because he couldn't fulfill his role in some of the traditional ways of the community. And every time he urged his wife that perhaps they get on with it in a different way, she'd have a terrible attack of migraine, and that would end the discussion.

So it went between us. She was trying to manipulate me. She apparently was succeeding in manipulating him. I couldn't tell whether my treatment was having any impact on her headache because I was basically fighting a possible drug dependency and fighting off patient manipulation. Somewhere out there were echoes I didn't quite hear—vague, indirect, quiet little sounds. We get so attuned to listening to our patients, to hearing their day-to-day complaints, that somehow, sometimes, we miss those faint but meaningful echoes.

One morning, I got a phone call from a clergyman who knew the family of my patient. It seemed that something had happened the night before. Perhaps it was a final, crushing despair, nobody knows exactly what happened or why, but my patient's husband had taken his life.

I never heard from her again.

29

THE FASHION DESIGNER'S NEW HEADACHE

From the moment I entered the examination room on her first visit to the Clinic, I observed that Annabelle Corbin was a woman who paid rather careful attention to her appearance. She was wearing a large, yellow, round hat with a white bow, one that I would not have been surprised to see Queen Elizabeth II wearing to the horse races at Royal Ascot. Her matching suit jacket and pants suggested a coordination that was not by mistake.

She extended her hand and firmly shook my hand as she said rather hurriedly, "How do you do? My name is Annabelle Corbin, and I sure as hell hope you can help me with my problem. I'm a very busy woman and, quite frankly, I haven't got time for this!" Realizing that she did not seem interested in continuing with a myriad of pleasantries, I said in return, "Nice to meet you. I will most certainly try. Now tell me about your headache."

When I first meet a headache patient, I like to start with an open-ended question that allows the patient to tell me what she thinks is the information that I need to know in order to help her. This serves several functions actually. First, it allows the patient to feel—rightly so, that she is being heard. So many patients that come to the Diamond Headache Clinic have felt ignored or dismissed by healthcare providers, and they have often become disillusioned with the medical community as a whole. Second, it truly does help me gather a great deal of the pertinent information that I need in order to make the correct diagnosis and formulate the proper treatment regimen, without the need for an exhaustive rapid-fire question session that could, in some instances, make the patient feel that she is being interrogated.

Annabelle Corbin proceeded to tell me that she had been having a constant, daily headache for the past 16 months. "I woke up one day, March 12 of last year to be exact, and the damn thing has not gone away since! I wake up with the headache, I go to bed with the headache." She continued to raise her voice and gesture with both hands for emphasis as she explained the details of her headache, how when she first woke with the headache that day in March she figured it was a minor issue that would pass. She had a bottle of ibuprofen[5] left over from when she had twisted her ankle two years prior, so she took the ibuprofen for two weeks before she finally called her primary care doctor for advice. "I was too busy to worry with it." She explained that she lives in New York City and works as a fashion designer, a job that "I absolutely love—it really is my life I suppose." She was 53 years old and had moved to New York from Georgia at the age of 19 "two years after I started to study design in Savannah I quit and moved to New York, and I worked my way up to where I am now." Where she was "now" was working as the lead fashion designer for one of the top fashion houses in New York. It was a very high-pressure, stressful position. She had been in that role for about two years. "It's not the job, if that's what you're thinking...I was the lead designer for a good six months before the headache started."

I asked her to tell me about headaches that she may have had before this headache episode. "None. Zero. I mean I had the occasional headache the morning after a night of drinking in my 20s, but that was never anything like this." During the interview I learned that she was the oldest of three children and was raised in the mountains of northern Georgia. "My goal from day one was to get out of that small town. I suppose that's why I like the energy of Manhattan— because it's so different from where I came." I was slightly surprised to learn that she was originally from Georgia, because I did not detect even the slightest southern accent from Annabelle Corbin.

Her headache was located in the forehead, which is known as the frontal region, with both sides affected. She noted the pain alternated between "dull and throbbing, depending on how severe it is." She said she typically woke with a level 4/10 headache, which felt like a dull pressure, but by the middle of

---

[5] A nonsteroidal anti-inflammatory drug (NSAID)

the afternoon it usually increased in intensity to a level 6-7/10 and was throbbing. She denied having sensitivity to light or sound, but she noted that she often felt nauseated with the more severe headache.

Annabelle Corbin's journey to the Diamond Headache Clinic was, in many ways, similar to that of many other patients that we see. She first saw her primary care physician, who told her that she had tension-type headache due to the stress of her job, and he prescribed a steroid for her to take for one week. When the headache did not improve with steroid, he referred her to a neurologist. "By that point I was already frustrated, as I had the headache for over a month and my work was beginning to suffer. She ordered an MRI, a spinal tap, and lots of blood tests, all of which were normal. I ended up with an even worse headache after the spinal tap—that headache was on top of my head and lasted for about a week. The only thing that made it better was to lay down. The minute I stood, the headache came back. Finally after a week I was back down to just one miserable headache."

The neurologist prescribed topiramate[6], which caused cognitive side effects that she tried to endure for about a month, "I couldn't come up with words—simple words that I—of all people—know, like fashion terms and such. It was unreal. I couldn't take it, and the headache didn't improve, so we switched to propranolol. I didn't have any problems with propranolol, but it made no difference in my headache. Finally I insisted we try BOTOX, because I had heard from a friend that it helped with her migraine. Nothing. I tried it three times, which took nine months in all, and there was no improvement in the headache. By now I was either leaving work early or missing work at least two days per week." She shared her frustration with the neurologist, who suggested she come to the Diamond Headache Clinic.

Annabelle Corbin's boss, the owner of the fashion house, expressed concern that the quality of her work had diminished in the past few months and

---

[6] An antiepileptic drug prescribed to prevent seizures. This drug is FDA-approved for the prevention of migraine.

suggested that she may need to consider taking a different position with less responsibility. "I persuaded her to give me one month to turn things around, and that's why I'm here. I need you to turn things around for me, otherwise I'm going to lose my job that means the world to me. Like I told you, I've worked my entire life to get here!" At that moment, she showed the first outward sign of vulnerability when her eyes welled up with tears, she bit her top lip, which was quivering, and she took a deep breath. She took a tissue from the desktop, matter of factly dabbed each eye in such a manner as to not smear her mascara, and then she paused and looked at me. "We will help you," I said, and I extended my hand; we shook hands, solidifying our partnership to work toward improving her headache.

We continued the office visit with a neurological exam, and once I had determined that her exam was completely normal, I sat down across from her. "You told me your primary care physician told you that you have tension-type headache. What did the neurologist tell you?" "She told me I had a combination of tension and migraine. I don't so much care what it is I have—I just want it gone!"

I explained to Annabelle Corbin that she had New Daily Persistent Headache (NDPH), which occurs when a patient without much of a headache history suddenly begins to have a headache that occurs every day. While the cause of NDPH is not known in many cases, often the headache starts in the setting of an infection or surgery. The most common cause of NDPH is thought to be the Epstein-Barr virus, which is the virus that causes the illness mononucleosis (mono). Plenty of patients with NDPH have never had mono, and as in the case of Annabelle Corbin, she did not recall having any symptoms of an infection around the time that her headache started. Sometimes NDPH has features of tension headache as well as migraine. "So in a way both of those doctors were correct." NDPH is known to be one of the more difficult headache conditions to treat, and its treatment is generally the same as that of migraine. I went on to discuss with Annabelle Corbin that her treatment would require she

216

be admitted to the Diamond Headache Inpatient Unit at Presence St. Joseph Hospital, and that her stay would likely be around one week. "One week?! I don't have one week to spend in the hospital! I only have one month to fix the mess that has become of my career, how can I spend one week of that here?" I reviewed with her the importance of breaking the cycle of headache that she was in, and I reminded her that strictly outpatient methods had so far given her very little, if any, improvement. "Ok, I'll give you one week—but not one day longer!"

The Diamond Headache Inpatient Unit has been the springboard for thousands of headache patients to return to an improved level of function. The unit has been deemed a center of excellence by several insurance companies due to the overall favorable results that patients achieve. Insurance companies, of course, often measure success in terms of dollars saved, and patients overall have significantly reduced ER visits for headache after having been admitted to the unit. Most importantly, however, patients' lives are improved.

Annabelle Corbin was admitted that very day and she began the medical treatment that I prescribed, which included intravenous dihydroergotamine (DHE)[7]. Since DHE can often cause nausea we administer it with an antinausea medication, in her case ondansetron (Zofran). When I saw her the next morning during rounds she reported to me that her headache was unchanged, and she admitted that she was worried that her headache was never going to improve. "Remember that I told you it may take a few days before you start to see much improvement," I said. She acknowledged that, yes, we had discussed that. "OK, let's just get me better!"

Throughout the next two days, she continued the DHE treatment every eight hours, and in between doses she participated in biofeedback training twice daily and attended classes on diet, relaxation, mindfulness, medications, among others. However, she was very hesitant to embrace biofeedback because she

---

[7] DHE is administered every eight hours for a total of nine doses. This protocol was developed by Neil Raskin, a headache specialist at the University of California San Francisco Medical Center.

refused to believe that stress and tension could be playing a role in her headache. Even after having the headache for 16 months, she held onto the belief that "I am plenty relaxed!" In fact, when I asked her in the office if she had ever felt that she was depressed or anxious, and if she was seeing a psychotherapist, she laughed and said, "I have neither the time nor the need to see a therapist!" Every patient admitted to the Diamond Inpatient Unit has at least one visit with a psychologist, and Annabelle Corbin was no exception. When I asked her about that visit, she reported that, to her surprise, the therapist gave her some good tips on relaxation and that she even planned to get referrals for therapists in her area. "I'm not sure if I'm quite ready to see my own therapist when I get home, but if it will help my headache like you say it will, I suppose I'm willing to give it a try."

By the end of the third day, Annabelle Corbin's headache was completely gone. When I saw her during morning rounds on her fourth day, she had packed her suitcase and was dressed in another matching suit, and she had a different, equally fashionable hat sitting next to her in the room. "I'm ready to get back to New York and to work! When can I go?" I explained to her that I wanted to keep her for one more day to ensure that, once the DHE treatment was complete, her headache did not return forcefully. I explained that the first 24 hours after DHE this is a possibility, "and you would prefer to be here in the hospital if it does, because in that event you will need another three days of DHE treatment." I assured her that she could go home the following day if her headache continued to be very low or gone. She agreed and took the opportunity to continue biofeedback treatment. I was later told by the nursing staff that Annabelle Corbin had befriended several of the other patients and even arranged for an impromptu fashion show that evening in the activities room. I suppose the other patients enjoyed experiencing a little bit of what a New York City fashion show was like.

During Annabelle Corbin's stay, in addition to DHE treatment, she was treated with intravenous orphenadrine (Norflex), which is a muscle relaxant, and

218

ketorolac (Toradol), which is an NSAID (anti-inflammatory). I started her on one daily prevention medication, a beta blocker called nebivolol (Bystolic)[8]. She would continue to take this daily to prevent the return of her headache to the previous frequency and severity. I explained that it would take a few weeks before we could really judge how well nebivolol was working, but since we were able to break the headache cycle with DHE I was confident nebivolol would have a good chance of helping.

The following morning Annabelle Corbin reported that she had been headache-free the entire day before, so we agreed that, yes it was time to go back to New York. I emphasized that I felt she should take the next few days off work, so that she would not feel as pressured to perform immediately. We compromised that she would take the following day, Friday, off, but she insisted she would be back at work first thing Monday morning. And she was.

When I saw Annabelle Corbin for her follow-up visit one month after she was discharged, she reported that her headache was much better. She had only had 1-2 minor headaches in the afternoon the past two weeks, but she was able to bring them under quick control with the nose spray version of DHE that I prescribed for her, Migranal. She had been utilizing biofeedback every day at work, and she felt this was allowing her to maintain a better balance in her day. She had even scheduled an appointment with one of the psychologists our team had provided for her. "The best part of it all, though, is that my job is secure again!"

I continued to see her every three months for about one year. At her one-year visit, she asked if she could stop taking nebivolol. Since she had virtually no headache for the previous six months, I agreed that she could try stopping it. In New Daily Persistent Headache, usually the headache eventually does go away, although it can take several years for this to happen. Treating with medications such as nebivolol seems to speed this along, and if it does not eliminate the headache entirely it lessens the frequency and severity so that the

---

[8] A beta blocker used in the treatment of cardiovascular disorders and in migraine prevention.

headache is more manageable. I instructed her to stop the medication but to keep her Migranal spray in the event that the headache returned. I asked her to notify me immediately if this happened, at which point she would restart nebivolol. I asked her to see me in six months either way. At the subsequent follow-up visit ,she continued to be headache-free even without taking nebivolol. It was safe to assume that, in the case of Annabelle Corbin, the NDPH was indeed a thing of her past. To this day, when I see fashion magazines at the supermarket, I wonder if Annabelle Corbin had some hand in designing the clothes featured on the cover. I smile and feel grateful that I was able to help her get back to the career she so loved.

30

A FINAL CASE—AND THOUGHT

I thought I would conclude this book with a discussion of migraine and how it affects people and some of the issues and generalizations of the problem, all as seen through the eyes of one migraine victim. Her views are, of course, quite individual, and yet they are not unusual. They have in them a feeling that is recognized or shared by a good many headache victims. Yvonne Brench is a woman of 37. She has three children. Her husband is a rising executive in an industrial firm in the Midwest. She has lived in various parts of the country, but she now lives in a very comfortable suburban home near a large city. She has a quick intelligence and a sharp, somewhat critical or skeptical mind. She has the singular fortune of considerable beauty, and she accepts it as naturally as her own skin. "I can remember in high school and college that if I wasn't asked out by at least four or five people on a Saturday night, I thought I was a failure, a washout." She couldn't go out on all of those dates, but she *expected* to be asked out by four or five different boys. "I didn't realize that so many girls—this was something I was terribly naïve about—that so many girls felt lucky if they had one date a week or even one date a month."

On the other hand, her life has had its difficulties. Her father was deeply disturbed by headaches; she believes now that they were migraine. Her brother is an alcoholic. Her oldest son is a victim of cerebral palsy. Her youngest child had a stomach malformation at birth that had to be corrected immediately by radical surgery. She has herself undergone serious surgery, most notably a hysterectomy. She has suffered from migraine headaches since she was nine years old. "What stands out in my mind is that I'd have a series of them," she said. "They almost invariably started on a Sunday. I never found out why. But I would be just violently ill. And the only thing I could do was go home and go to bed."

Interestingly, she remembers having the headaches in her teenage years, but they are not the predominant memory of those times. "In the dating period, I can remember saying, 'I have to go home early,' when I really didn't have early hours at home," she said. "I could be at a basketball game; I could be at the movies; I could be any place, and I would have to get up and leave and come home. There was only one place for me and that place was in bed—the pain was so great." And yet it was the breathless popularity that she enjoyed in those years that sticks in her mind. She does not feel that she suffered from ill-health in her last three years in high school, and she remembers mostly that she dedicated herself to having fun, and achieving her goal, when she was in college.

Her migraine seemed to mount in intensity shortly after she got married. She would get an aura that would give her a warning of the headache. "I'd walk down a street, or drive, and look at a sign and three letters would be missing. It's not that they looked overlapped," she said, "but I just couldn't see three letters on the sign." In addition, her tongue would become numb, starting on the side where the headache would occur.

The aura provided her with a warning—not to take medicine to head off the migraine (for she had no such medicine then), but to get home and get to bed. "I knew I had only 15 minutes to get home. Coffee, lunches, anything—I'd get up and leave and get in the car and drive home as fast as I could." In the early years of her marriage, she lived on the outskirts of Boston and often drove into the city. "If I went into Boston, I wouldn't be able to get home, if only because of the complicated traffic problems." The pain would strike her while she was still on the road, and the pain would be almost crippling. Her solution was to stay off the road and not go into Boston. So the migraine was interfering somewhat with her life even then.

She began keeping a diary and a calendar to see if there was a cycle to her migraine pains that would free her to go out on certain days. Many migraine patients do the same thing. But she built more into it than a time factor. "I

222

wanted to know why. Was there something that would cause the migraine on some days and not on others?" At that time, she didn't know of migraine personality studies and that the migraine victim often possesses stress factors and a sense of responsibility more acute than those of other people. She didn't know quite what to look for so she wrote down the most immediate cause of great stress—whether the children had been squabbling, whether she and her husband had a fight or didn't have a fight ("no turmoil, no fight with Bob"), even whether he'd gone out of town. "I began to think it was because Bob was traveling so much that I had a migraine," she said. Now she knows better, but she is still pulled by the possibility and by the coincidence of his travel and her migraine. "Because he went on a trip not too long ago, and the first day he was out of town, I had a migraine," she said. About the only thing the calendar told her is what her body told her: she'd most certainly have migraine about the time of her period or ovulation or both. "If I ovulated and went into Boston that day, well, I knew that I wouldn't be able to get home." Her life began to revolve around that calendar and the pain that it might predict.

Her calendar would help her eliminate the complications of an attack of migraine. For instance, she would not drive a car the day the headache would strike. But the calendar could not eliminate the pain of the migraine which began to strike more and more often. It was not timed solely, any longer, to her period—not that this was new or unusual. She knew she began having migraine at the age of nine, but she didn't have her first period until she was a sophomore in high school. So there had to be a period of five or six years in which she had the pain but not the period.

So she began looking for other cause of the pain—what we might call the triggers of the migraine. She noticed that the headaches seemed more acute when there was a change of seasons—into spring and into fall. She came to believe that the smoke of burning leaves, so pleasant to most of us, was triggering her migraine in the fall. There was nothing she could do about spring—she suspected pollen or the effluvia of budding trees and plants. But that made her think of dust in the air, and she had the furnace and the heating and cooling system in her home checked to see whether it was circulating some malevolent element (it wasn't). She did conclude that perfume was a trigger and she not only avoided using it but tried to avoid those environments where it was in heavy use. This eliminates not only an awful lot of parties but a good many beauty parlors. ("My friends are very protective of me, to the extent that they will not wear perfume because I can't tolerate it," she said.) She found also that she could not drink beer or red wine and very little alcoholic spirits of any kind. And on one of her stays in the hospital—for her hysterectomy, I believe—she was told that she had a very high level of estrogen in her system. "The gynecologist showed me charts for the different levels of estrogen and mine was so high that it wasn't even included on the charts." As we've seen from earlier cases, estrogen is implicated in the triggering of migraine in a great many women.

She went to the doctor, of course. She went to doctor after doctor after doctor. None of them, she feels, satisfactorily attacked the headaches. She feels that they tended to prescribe painkillers and tell her to learn to live with the problem. The painkillers became her crutch.

But she felt that they were not helping. "The painkillers camouflaged the problem; they didn't cure it," she said. They were effective, in her experience, for about four hours. When the four hours were up, I was deathly sick all over again because the migraine pains didn't just last for four hours. They would last from 18 to 24 hours." The only way to handle continuing pain is to take the painkiller continuously. "And I didn't want to live my life at the red-label level"—the red label warning of the presence of a very powerful drug. So she looked for another doctor, and yet another and another.

She insists today they would do nothing but prescribe a painkiller. They would look no further for the cause of the headache than to say "it's just nerves." This annoyed her; the suggestion of "nerves" still does. "First you have to live with the pain," she said. "Then you visit a doctor and he makes you feel

224

like a psychosomatic nut. Many doctors have no patience, no sympathy, no understanding of what you're going through. Physically you're racked with pain; whether it is brought on by nerves or anything else, you're still racked with pain.

"The only time a doctor will recognize the pain of a migraine victim is if he has a migraine himself or if he knows another doctor who has migraine. And then it's because that Dr. So-and-So had to shut down his practice for a while because of a migraine or cluster headache. That's really something—when a doctor closes down his practice because of a migraine, now *that's* something. The trouble is, I've only met two doctors who've known other doctors who had migraine." And both of them were deep into headaches as a medical specialty.

That's another thing that bothered Yvonne Brench; the doctors she met who were in general or family practice either didn't know there were specialists in the treatment of headache or neglected to pass that information on to the patient. To a certain extent, I can understand that. It is a probative posture for a physician not to recommend going to a specialist, if only because of the added cost to the patient, unless and until he knows that he, the family physician, can't do anything more for the patient. And a great many family physicians feel that they can offer the headache patient all that a specialist can. Certainly they can handle the cases involving a casual or passing headache. It is only the most difficult cases that, justifiably, are passed on to the headache specialist. And certainly the drugs and the knowledge for treating headaches, even migraine and cluster, are available to the internist or the doctor in family practice. There is nothing exclusive in this. In fact, the headache specialist doesn't want it to be exclusive; he wants to share his information. In addition, managed care, which has taken over the cost of treating headaches by the medical insurance companies, makes it most difficult to recommend a headache specialist.

That's one of the functions of the National Headache Foundation. It not only opens its membership to interested doctors, but it publishes a newsletter with articles from all over the world on scientific investigation and clinical experience with headache. It is, in fact, the only lay publication in America that is devoted exclusively to a symptom. Further, the National Headache Foundation, headquartered in Chicago, accepts laypeople as well as doctors as members. Headache sufferers can receive helpful information, including a list of doctor members, by visiting the NHF website at www.headaches.org.

If there is any advantage that the headache specialist has over the internist or the family practitioner, it is in the range of experience and the depth of insight. It is the same advantage that any specialist in medicine possesses. The headache specialist tends to see patients as individuals with individual problems, where the family practitioner or the internist—overburdened with patients with seemingly more urgent pains—tends to accept headache victims as being of a single class, usually one with "nerves" as a common problem.

There is, perhaps, one other difference: the headache specialist will stay with the problem of the patient until he or she solves it or at least reduces it to manageable proportions. The headache specialist knows that a pain in the head that a patient has had for many, many years is not going to disappear overnight. You can overcome the pain with a painkiller, but that is a temporary expedient. The pain will return when the impact of the painkiller is ended. To find and attack the cause of the pain may take several months or even several years. But the headache specialist will stay with the problem when often the primary care provider—the internal medicine or family medicine physician, nurse practitioner, or physician assistant—is likely to give up on the headache problem to treat patients he or she thinks (often mistakenly) are more seriously ill.

In the case of Yvonne Brench, the failure of treatment through the first line of medical help, which was the family practitioner, coincided with increased stresses and responsibilities in her life. She was determined to be a good and conscientious mother to her son, despite his problem with cerebral palsy. She was not going to abandon him to general care; she was not going to deliver him to an institution "I always encouraged him to live as normal a life as possible," she said. She was determined to be there with him, to make sure nobody said to him, "No, you can't do that because you have cerebral palsy." Her reason was simple: "To me, he was my baby and I always wanted to encourage him to do as much as he could. They told me that he was a complete cerebral palsy victim and would never be able to do anything for himself. It wasn't that I didn't believe them, it was that I wanted to do the best job that I could." The result: the boy goes to a public school; he gets on a school bus by himself; he functions in a normal world despite his handicap. The determined attention of his mother to the goal of normalcy was perhaps the greatest gift of his life.

At the same time, Yvonne Brench's life had other stresses. There was the problem with her youngest child—the malrotation of the infant's stomach. There was the uprooting of the family and moving it to a new location; she recognizes that this may have caused a stress situation—a visceral objection to the move—but she points out that it also came in the autumn. "And that may have been a factor" in the rise in incidence of her headache pain. And finally there was the possibility that her youngest daughter, now seven, was already showing signs of having migraine. "Whenever she comes in from play—perfectly normal play, with everything going beautifully—and says, 'I have a headache and have to go to bed,' that reminds me of exactly what I did when I was a child," she said.

Beyond all this, she drove herself in outside work. She was in volunteer work. She worked on the board of the local community center. She worked for the Republican Women's Club and rose to a responsible position. She went to work for a local congressman and accepted a menial position in his campaign. If there was a group needing help, she joined it. "My suburb is a great opening ground for such activities," she said. "I tried them all."

The headaches grew worse, the pain became more intense, and the total impact became almost crippling. For the migraine not only devastated her with pain but left her racked with nausea. "To the point where I was hospitalized twice, and when we moved from New England to here, they wanted to hospitalize me again because I was so deathly ill," she said.

Bit by bit, her condition deteriorated. Nothing seemed to improve it, no doctor, no treatment. Several years ago, the pain and the general torment became so continuous that she barely could get out of bed from one attack before the net attack would hit her and send her back to bed. She'd been sick in bed for a month and a half before she first came to see me. She was not capable of walking alone into my office. She needed assistance in whatever she did.

In that first meeting, we carried out the usual procedure: a physical exam, a searching interview, a discussion of what might be done and what had to be done, and a first step in the discipline toward reaching the goal. We gave her some emergency treatment and prescribed a medication which we thought would be helpful until her next visit. Later she was to tell me that she was in a state of euphoria by the time she got home. She thought it was the medication. I thought it was the aftereffect of migraine that some such victims undergo. Now she believes it was the effect of being freed from pain for the first time in six weeks.

If that sounds miraculous—well, don't believe it. There were no miracles in the treatment of Yvonne Brench. Each step had to be taken slowly, with a searching sense of what was right as well as what was effective. There was, as always, the exploration of what drugs in what quantities through what routes of administration would work best. Bit by bit, we got the headaches under control. When they eased off, as they seemed to do in certain cycles, she'd reduce her consumption of the medicine. When they came on hard again, she'd increase it. And with all this, she tried to control the stress factors in her own life. She decided which of her many tasks—volunteer and otherwise—were important to her, and she dropped the rest. Her family was important and, she decided, politics was important. So she's kept up her involvement with politics along with her family imperatives.

The result is that her headaches are vastly reduced, she is no longer confined to bed, she is able to function normally in life, but her headaches are not completely gone. She still gets a migraine once a month—usually late in the

228

month. ("I mark it on my calendar," she said.) She also gets the headache in what seem to be unusual circumstances, either of stress or change of environment. She and the family went to Cape Cod for a summer vacation a year or so ago. She had a headache of intense proportions shortly after getting there, and then it cleared up. When they drove home—it *was* a long drive—she had a headache of intense proportions when she got back. So she is not headache-free. She is merely in better control of them than ever before. She controls her life now, instead of having the headaches—the calendar of pain—control it.

Now that you know a good deal about Yvonne Brench, I thought you would be interested in what she has to say about the issues and details associated with her complaint.

On the pain of migraine: "I think every chronic headache victim, migraine or otherwise, probably feels that there's a tumor there. You think that anything that severe—you can't describe it...I thought I had a brain tumor. That has to be the ultimate pain." (Doctor's note: It isn't.)

"If you have that much pain, there has to be a reason for it. It's not because you're nervous or upset. It has to be something organic that's causing this. I've gone through childbirth. I've gone through major surgery. I'd rather go through either one or both than have a migraine. The pain is that great and that crippling, to the point where you cannot function, you cannot move. It's unbelievable, the pain. When I had the hysterectomy, the doctor was a personal friend and he was very understanding and he said, 'You're going to have a tough pull when you come out of surgery. There's going to be a lot of pain, but we'll take care of you'—meaning he'd give me painkillers. But I only took one painkiller after surgery. My doctor said that he'd never before had a patient who could come out of surgery like that and take only one painkiller. The simple fact was that I was so inured to pain from my migraine headaches that the pain of surgery, the pain of a hysterectomy, was nothing in comparison to it."

On the threat of death: "What doctors tell you, in different words, is that headaches are not fatal. I suppose this is why their concern is not so great. I've been told that I'll never die from migraine." (Doctor's note: As we've seen from a previous chapter, migraine can cause death through the disruption and harassment of the family—and it can inspire thought of death, through suicide, in its victims.)

"I've said many times that I would rather die than continue going through this for the rest of my life. I told one doctor that although I would never personally contemplate suicide, I would gladly welcome death over the continuing pain of migraine. The pain—it's hard for me to describe it now that I've been removed from its constant nature for a year or two. Except that when I do have a migraine now, I think, 'Oh my God! How did I ever live through it, day in and day out!'"

On the trait of brilliance in the migraine personality: "That's supposed to compensate for the pain. They always used to tell me that Tolstoy had migraine, and Freud had migraine, and Darwin, and Chopin. As if all that was going to wipe away my migraine. Isn't it interesting that all these brilliant, talented men had migraine and they could nothing to help themselves? You have to search hard for anybody in medicine who can tell you anything more about migraine except, 'Take this painkiller and go home and go to bed.' The first thing the doctors tell you is 'You're high strung. And you're intelligent.' So I'm intelligent. I've met a lot of people who are a lot more intelligent than I am, and they don't have migraine. If they're so smart, why don't they have migraine?"

On other traits of the migraine personality: "I've never felt that I matched the migraine personality, although many doctors have told me that I do. 'You're high strung and fastidious and intelligent,' they say. Well, I am *not* fastidious. Really I'm not. They say, 'You must have the cleanest house. You spend all your time cleaning the house.' I keep saying, 'Would you like to come over and see my house? I'll show you how fastidious I am.' The only thing is there are incidents which make me think there is something to all this. I've heard about the chair in Dr. Diamond's office—the chair that he keeps out of place to see if the patient will move it back into place and thus give a hint as to whether he's a migraine personality. Well I've never been put to that test, and I never thought I'd move that chair because I think I'm a little different and that I deviate from the formula. In that I am not fastidious. But I can remember going to a furniture show with a friend and walking through a display with a four-piece sectional sofa with the various pieces out of alignment. And I couldn't stand it. I had to stop and go over and put those pieces all together in the right way. There must have been 100 people in that room—we were going through in a large crowd—and not one of them particularly cared about the sofa being out of alignment. But I just couldn't stop myself. I had to go over and make everything just right."

On being a driven personality: "I've heard this about migraine victims and I've studied it in myself. And I think I'm driven by anything that I decide to take on, anything that's part of my personal goals. But anything that's assigned to me, that people think is my 'duty,' I'm not driven or dedicated about. On the other hand, if I tell you that I'm personally going to do something, you can rest assured that it's going to be done well and properly."

On the traits of migraine victims: "I think more often than not you'll find that migraine people are extremely analytical, almost more so than being perfectionists. We always try to figure out 'Why?' If somebody makes a remark that's bothersome to Bob, my husband, he'll just overlook it and forget about it. But if they say it to me, I'll remember it. I'll go home and I'll think about it and say, 'Why? What precipitated that? Was I obnoxious?' I think you find a lot of migraine people are like that. If they keep a diary, they don't want to know just what occurred or when a headache occurred, they want to know why."

On the "nerve syndrome" of migraine patients: "The more I think about migraine, the less I think that nerves or psychology or any of that matters. I think maybe they aggravate it, but I don't think they create it. If it were just a matter of nerves, then the whole world would be migraine sufferers. When my last child was born, she had a malrotation of the stomach and intestines. They were tuned 90 degrees, and she had to have surgery when she was only a few weeks old. The surgery was so severe that the doctors said whether she lived or died would be decided on the operating table. I was emotionally torn. I was incapable of functioning. Yet I never had a headache in that entire period. All that time, not knowing whether she was going to live or die, all during her recovery in the hospital, all during the difficult time when we took her home— all this and I never once suffered a migraine headache. I feel that if it was nerve-oriented, it would have come out at that time. But I did not have a migraine until my second period after the birth.

"When my oldest child was born, it was a very difficult birth. He had cerebral palsy, and he was not expected to live. A minister was called in. My husband, who was in the service then, was notified by telegram that his son was about to die. I was alone with the problem, and yet I never had a migraine at that time. There was a significant problem of stress, and yet it didn't cause a migraine problem then. So you have to wonder when a doctor tells you that migraine is just a matter of nerves." (Doctor's note: In fairness, migraine is a much more complex matter than "nerves" alone.)

As is suggested by these examples, the hormonal balance of the female migraine victim may also be very influential in the incidence and intensity of her attack. During and just after pregnancy, the secretion of certain female hormone changes and, perhaps because of this, the migraine attacks lessen. Yvonne Brench's experiences indicate that stress or "nerves" alone are not enough to induce a migraine attack. But this doesn't mean that stress or "nerves" won't contribute to triggering a migraine attack when the other factors, such as hormonal balance, make the victim susceptible to it. In short, when all the complex factors involved in migraine come together, stress or "nerves" may still be one of the factors involved in it. At least in some patients.

"I felt I was close to a nervous breakdown during the last crisis in which my youngest child was so grievously stricken. But I've since concluded

232

that I don't think I could have a nervous breakdown—not during a period when migraine is present. Because the migraine is a warning signal. It tells me to stop. Not only does it 'tell' me that, but it leaves me totally incapacitated. That's the only thing that will make me give in. Unless it's something like that, I just won't stop what I'm doing, what I need to do, I can't—I won't let anything upset me then. That's why I think the migraine puts a brake on the tendency to go until you break down."

On the "high wall" of the migraine victim: "This one thing I've learned—the migraine victim will never spontaneously discuss headaches with somebody in the 'normal' world. We'll pass information to each other but not to you, the normal, everyday person we encounter in life. This must have something to do with the 'weaknesses' of somebody who is laid low with 'only' a headache. We'll all talk about our operations—I'll talk about my hysterectomy in great detail. We all do it. But it has to be a very, very serious thing before I let down and talk about my migraine. I can remember one friend with whom I worked long and hard hours on a particular project that was close to both of us—politics. There were times when we were under a tremendous amount of stress. And yet she never knew that I suffered from migraine pain. And I never knew until later that she did, too. For she never told me, and I never told her, of the problem that bothered us both."

On the common conception of migraine victims: "It absolutely incenses me when someone on television says, 'I think I'll have a migraine after this situation.' I sit there and get so angry. Because if you really have migraine, you don't say that. Not if you care about those around you. I mean, if I have a tremendous fight with Bob, I don't go off and say, 'I think I'll have a migraine.' If I'm having a migraine, I won't tell anybody that I'm having a migraine. I try to force myself through the situation. I try to continue on in as normal a life as long as I can and do whatever I'm obligated to do. I don't want to go to bed and be sick. I simply go to bed as the last resort."

This is not the end. It is merely a time to pause. We have heard the voices, now we shall listen to the echoes.

But if there is anything that might have been learned to this moment, it is that headache pain is common but not simple. It demands much of the doctor—in insight, knowledge, and understanding. It demands much of the patient—a perspective on pain that is sometimes hard to express. With the combination of the two and the high purpose of medicine, the pain of headache might be reduced or even erased.

31

POSTSCRIPT

Update in the Treatment of Headache

As we noted in the preface to this edition, many of the histories related here are several years old. They reveal the processes that we go through to investigate the cause of headache and the methods we use to develop a treatment plan to help handle each individual's headaches.

Medical science has continued to advance since many of these patients were first treated. Newer techniques have been developed to study the body and our understanding of what cause headaches has progressed. With this we have found many new treatments for the various kinds of headaches. We have updated some of the diagnostic studies and medication regimens to more closely reflect the treatments that are used today.

Pain such as headache remains a subjective symptom. As a result there is no tool available to physicians to tell us what kind of pain a patient suffers from nor how severe that pain is. Many techniques, including blood tests, MRIs, and MRAs have been used to help try to find a way to test for specific types of headache. However, none of these tests at present provides an accurate marker to make a diagnosis of migraine, cluster, or tension-type headache.

Magnetic Resonance Imaging (MRI)

The diagnosis of headache still rests on taking a careful history, performing a thorough examination, and, if necessary, doing such tests as CT scans and blood work. These tests are performed not so much to make a diagnosis, but rather to make sure that a more serious or organic problem is not responsible for the headache and neurologic symptoms that a headache sufferer experiences. One of the best tests that science has developed to help us is the *MRI*. It is also known as *nuclear magnetic resonance* (*NMR*). These terms refer to the ability to take a picture of the brain by looking at how the atoms in the brain respond to the effects of radio waves within a large magnet. Scientists discovered years ago that every chemical responds a little bit differently to the effects of radio waves when placed in a strong magnetic field; literally, a fingerprint exists for each chemical in nature. This same type of technique applied on a larger scale allows us to take a picture of the brain. Each section of the brain and organic problems within the brain, such as tumors, cysts, blood clots, scar tissue from a stroke, or even the plaques seen in multiple sclerosis, produce their own unique picture on the MRI scan. MRI has helped us to investigate and determine the source of several patients' problems.

A few years back, for example, we saw a young woman who had been to many doctors before coming to us for her headaches. What was most distressing to this woman was not the pain, since it was relatively mild, but rather the fact that she experienced severe nausea and vomiting every several weeks. The nausea and vomiting lasted for days at a time and, as a result, the woman needed to be hospitalized and given intravenous fluids. All of our exams, tests, and treatments proved fruitless in explaining the cause of her problem. Finally, we used the MRI, which unfortunately revealed a small tumor located in a portion of the brain called the brain stem. This portion of the brain is the control center for all of the nerves of the head—it controls vital functions such as blood pressure, heart rate, and our breathing pattern, and it carries all the messages from the body to the brain and back to the body. In addition, there is a small group of cells that exists in the brain stem, and when these cells are stimulated in a certain fashion, they cause a person to become nauseated and to vomit. The MRI enabled us to find the cause of this patient's problem.

In another patient who was rather elderly, we thought a stroke she had suffered was causing some deterioration of nervous system functioning. Her previous tests had included a CT scan, brain scan, and even angiograms of the small blood vessels of the brain. All were normal, but her MRI scan revealed a small area of scar tissue that would have occurred as a result of a stroke right in

236

the area of the brain that controlled the specific functions that had failed in her case. Besides using this test to look for these types of problems, an MRI may also be helpful if a person cannot have a CT scan because they are severely allergic to the X-ray dye we need to use, or they are susceptible to radiation sickness in which the exposure to X-rays makes them very ill. The magnetic resonance image does not use any type of radiation to make its picture. Instead, it uses magnets and radio waves which are similar to the type of radio waves that bring us the sound on our radios. Moreover, the test causes no pain. The most difficult part of the test is the need to lie very still in the rather small opening between the magnets.

Tricyclic Antidepressants

Research into brain chemistry has shown us that in depression, chemicals called neurotransmitters become depleted. These chemicals—serotonin, norepinephrine, and others—are necessary for the nervous system to communicate the nerve impulses properly from one cell to the next. When these chemicals are not present, the nervous system cannot perform its functions normally. Depending on which areas of the brain are affected, this can cause disturbances of sleep, appetite, and memory; behavior may also be affected. Pain can result from this as well and may be the reason why patients with depression have chronic headache. Interestingly, in migraine headache, this depletion of neurotransmitters also appears to occur with each migraine headache attack. It is for this reason that the antidepressant drugs may help to treat migraine headaches as well as depression. This benefit in migraine is unrelated to a person being depressed.

Accountant James Michaels, a 52-year-old patient of the Clinic, suffered from both depression and migraine. He had been given different antidepressants which helped his depression, yet never seemed to help his migraines. Conversely, other drugs, including some antidepressants, helped his migraines, yet did little to help his depression. Through careful observation, we

237

eventually found an antidepressant which helped both his migraines and his depression. We used a medication called protriptyline (Vivactil). Like amitriptyline, this medicine is also an antidepressant, but unlike amitriptyline, it is not a sedative. Rather, it is more stimulating, so it needs to be taken during the daytime. It has this effect because it works on different neurotransmitters from those affected by amitriptyline. This patient's case not only helps illustrate the difference between depression and migraine, but it also shows the significance of considering why certain drugs may benefit one person and not another.

The slight difference in the lack of neurotransmitters indicates the importance of trying different medicines within the same class of medication to find a successful resolution in combating headache problems. Important work by Dr. Howard Fields, a noted pain researcher from the University of California at San Francisco, has shown that these drugs, by themselves, also have the ability to relieve the pain in a fashion similar to the pain-relieving analgesics. If these drugs had been developed today rather than some 30 years ago, they might be known as analgesics and not antidepressants.

Beta Blockers

Beta blockers have revolutionized the treatment of migraine since their first use in the United States in the mid-1970s. There are a number of these medications available to treat migraine. First developed to treat heart disease, such as disorders of cardiac rhythm and angina pectoris, as well as high blood pressure, it was soon discovered that beta blockers could be used to prevent migraine headaches. Propranolol (Inderal), a beta blocker, performs many activities that may contribute to its efficacy in migraine prevention including (1) preventing dilation of the cranial arteries because it blocks the beta receptors; (2) blocking the platelet aggregation induced by the catecholamines (any of various amines that function as hormones or neurotransmitters or both); and (3) decreasing the ability of platelets to adhere to the capillary wall. Research studies and clinical experience have shown that propranolol is the safest and most effective tool that

238

doctors have available to prevent migraine headaches. The long-acting form of propranolol, Inderal LA, can conveniently and safely be taken once a day for effective prevention.

Alpha Agonists

Other drugs work on these same type of receptors in the blood vessels to prevent migraine. But unlike the beta blockers, these are called alpha agonists; that is, they stimulate the alpha receptors and may keep the blood vessels under control and prevent migraine in a manner similar to the beta blockers. Clonidine (Catapres) is an alpha agonist. In some European countries it is considered the drug of choice to treat migraine headache. This drug is important to migraine treatment for several reasons. First, migraineurs who also have diabetes may be unable to take Inderal because it could hide a low blood sugar reaction from too much insulin. Catapres, however, will not mask this sort of reaction. Second, women who are continuing to get severe migraine after menopause may also be able to control the hot flashes that occur as the amount of estrogen decreases in the body. If these women take an estrogen preparation to control their hot flashes, this can increase the migraines. But with Catapres they might be able to control their migraines and their hot flashes, yet eliminate the excess estrogen from their system. Third, many migraine patients are susceptible to the effect of foods that contain the chemical tyramine. Tyramine is found in foods that are fermented, such as cheese, herring, liver, and citrus fruits. While it is a naturally occurring product of the fermentation of protein, tyramine can bring on migraine headaches in some people. This particular effect of tyramine—the one that can cause migraine—may be inhibited by Catapres.

Calcium Channel Blockers

The calcium channel blockers work on the blood vessels to treat both migraine headache and cluster headache. These drugs are very interesting since they may also have actions on brain cells to prevent the effects of lack of oxygen. Even

239

before a migraine attack strikes with its pain, the blood vessels may be experiencing a narrowing which may cause the brain to become starved for oxygen. This type of effect may be what causes the visual and other neurologic disturbances which occur as the prodrome to or warning of a migraine attack. Part of this effect of insufficient oxygen on the brain cells is brought about by the flow of calcium ions into the brain cells. This same kind of effect on the flow of calcium into these cells appears to be responsible for the action of the calcium channel blockers on the brain's blood vessels. And, by working on the blood vessels, it appears to help prevent both migraine and cluster headaches.

Many of the drugs that work with migraine may make use of this mechanism to prevent the headaches. Research has shown that cyproheptadine (Periactin), which is a first-generation antihistamine, and the antidepressants, such as Elavil, have calcium channel blocking action. These two medicines are not as potent as others in blocking this action. However, there are several others that appear to be very potent. Verapamil and nifedipine are both available in the United States and are used to help prevent migraine. Several other drugs have been used by our clinic in research in the treatment of migraine and cluster headache. Both U.S. and European studies have shown flunarizine and nimodipine to be very promising in this respect.

Unfortunately, it takes a very long time to study these medicines to ensure that they are useful and that they are going to be safe for people to take without risk of serious complications. In the United States, this research work is monitored by the Food and Drug Administration (FDA), which must approve all drugs before they are sold to the public. It also takes a long time for these medicines to work in the body to prevent the headaches. In migraine, it may take at least two weeks before any change is seen. Furthermore, the change might not include a reduction in the number of headaches, but rather the patients may stop experiencing their warning prodromes. In some patients, it can take as long as two or three months before the headaches begin to subside. Unfortunately, this can be very frustrating for the patient as well as the doctor.

240

Cluster headaches also are treated with medications other than these calcium channel blockers. Part of the decision in the treatment of cluster depends on the type of cluster headache the patient suffers from.

We divide cluster into several disorders. As we have noted previously, the most common variety of cluster headaches occur as what we call "episodic" cluster headache. With this type of cluster, the attacks occur daily for anywhere from several weeks to several months, and then there is a long pain-free remission that can extend for many years in some patients. For these patients, medicines such as the corticosteroids, triptans, and oxygen work very well.

Other cluster sufferers, predominantly women, have the cluster headache variant that responds specifically to indomethacin.

The last group of cluster sufferers is perhaps the most unfortunate because although they get headaches similar to the episodic variety, these patients do not have any long pain-free remission; they may get the cluster headaches daily for years on end. Drugs such as steroids could cause potentially disastrous consequences if they were taken for this amount of time. So for these patients, we need medicines that are safe and effective for long-term treatment. The calcium channel blockers are only one treatment alternative. Lithium carbonate (Eskalith) is one of the best medications to treat cluster headache of the chronic variety. It was developed to treat bipolar disorder, yet cluster patients rarely suffer from this disorder. It still remains the drug of choice to treat chronic cluster headache.

A small percentage of cluster sufferers fail at first to respond to these medicines, but if they do, they are likely to respond to them if they first undergo the histamine desensitization procedure described in an earlier chapter. It is now available in a once-a-day long-acting form which makes it convenient for the patient. Alpha agonists and other drugs work on these same types of problems.

Antiepileptic Drugs (AEDs)

241

We also prescribe antiepileptic medications to prevent migraine. Topiramate (Topamax) and Sodium Valproate (Depakote) are both FDA-approved for the prevention of migraine. Each medication is available in twice-daily or once-daily dosing. Side effects from topiramate include cognitive effects (such as difficulty with word-finding) and weight loss. Sodium valproate can cause weight gain, hair loss, and tremor. In addition, levetiracetam (Keppra) and gabapentin (Neurontin) can be used to prevent the frequency and severity of migraine.

There are many other treatments for aborting and for preventing the various types of headaches from occurring. To cover them all would be far beyond the scope of information that we are able to cover here.

32

POSTCRIPT II

Inpatient Care for the Difficult Patient

The use of an inpatient setting for the treatment of chronic headache disorders
has become an accepted and validated medical practice. Hospitalized patients
can indeed benefit from individualized therapy, careful monitoring, and a
comprehensive treatment program that may draw on staff and services not
usually available to outpatients.

Yet, with the current trend of escalating health care costs, increasing
emphasis has been placed on outpatient treatment for a variety of medical
problems including headaches. Inpatient care, compared with outpatient
treatment, is costlier for the patient, employer, and insurance industry.
Nevertheless, hospitalization is necessary for those headache patients who have
failed to respond to outpatient therapy. In short, patients with intractable
headaches may respond best to inpatient therapy followed by careful outpatient
follow-up. The insurance industry recognized this several years ago, thanks
largely to the painstaking work of the Diamond Headache Clinic. Several
insurance companies have deemed the Diamond Inpatient Unit a center of
excellence, due to its truly multidisciplinary approach to the treatment of
headache and its role in improved outcomes for patients. One metric that
insurance companies monitor, for example, is emergency department (ED)
visits. Patients who have been treated at the Diamond Inpatient Unit have
significantly fewer ED visits for headache after treatment. This underscores the
improved quality of life, in addition to lower future healthcare costs, that these
patients enjoy.

Patient selection for admission to a headache unit, such as the Diamond
Headache Clinic's inpatient unit at Presence St. Joseph Hospital in Chicago,
must follow strict criteria. Certain requirements have been established, and one

or more must be met before a patient is admitted to the unit. The criteria for admission are as follows:

- Prolonged, unrelenting headache, with associated symptoms, such as nausea and vomiting, that, if allowed to continue, would pose a further threat to the patient's welfare.
- Status migraine (migraine headache lasting more than 36 hours).
- Dependence on analgesics, caffeine, narcotics, barbiturates, or tranquilizers.
- Habituation to triptans; when patients who have taken triptans daily stop taking them, a rebound headache is the result.
- Pain that is accompanied by serious adverse reactions or complications from therapy; continued use of such therapy aggravates pain.
- Pain that occurs in the presence of significant medical disease; appropriate treatment of headache symptoms aggravates or induces further illness.
- Chronic cluster that is unresponsive to treatment.
- Treatment requiring copharmacy with drugs that may cause a drug interaction and necessitating careful observation within a hospital environment such as monoamine oxidase (MAO) inhibitors and beta blockers.
- Patients whose headaches have a probable organic cause and who require appropriate consultations and perhaps neurosurgical intervention.

There are relatively few patients who need inpatient care for pain that does not occur daily. These patients may have intractable pain complaints, but they may not have been given effective medication on an initial visit to a physician. In most cases, the pain is not completely relieved by analgesics, or if pain relief is achieved, it is a short duration. These patients seldom require hospitalization. The notable exception is the patient who has been using large quantities of over-the-counter analgesics containing caffeine or other sympathomimetic drugs on a daily basis.

Inpatient care if often useful when complications arise due to combination therapies or other medical problems. A large number of medical conditions may complicate the treatment of headache. A careful history and physical evaluation are, therefore, imperative. Careful evaluation of the patient may indicate the need for inpatient treatment to achieve the required balance in treating the headache problem as well as the other medical problems which exist concurrently. If the headache unit has been established in a large hospital, consultations with other specialists, if warranted, are facilitated. A cooperative effort among staff members ensures optimal, multidisciplinary, and continuous care of the hospitalized patient.

Often, coexisting disease processes may aggravate the headache problem. A treatment program for other medical problems—such as some antibiotics used for infections—may also increase the headaches. Alternative treatment programs for the medical problems may be considered in these cases. In still other cases, the proposed therapy for headaches may complicate the other medical conditions. Psychological factors are frequently severe enough to require an integration of focused psychological care with appropriate management of the headache problem.

Most patients requiring admission to our inpatient unit are ingesting excessive quantities of analgesic agents or triptans. The triptans that are used to abort headache attacks may cause rebound headaches when taken more than twice per week. Aspirin or NSAID intake on a daily basis may induce significant blood loss through minor gastric bleeding. Massive hemorrhage may occur if the dose and frequency of ingestion are considerable. Other side effects of excessive aspirin ingestion include peptic ulcers, skin rash, asthma, or aggravation of persisting liver disease. Excessive use of NSAIDs can lead to stomach ulcers as well as kidney disease. Medication overuse headache can develop when more than 10 doses of opioids such as hydrocodone or oxycodone are taken per month.

Therefore, carefully monitored withdrawal from previous analgesics is the first step toward controlling the patient's headache pain and, of course, controlling the pain is the primary goal of the inpatient headache treatment program. As with every aspect of the program, the approach to pain control is multidisciplinary. The first step is detoxification. This generally occurs during the first week of treatment when the patient is withdrawn from previous analgesic medications, including narcotics and barbiturates, and from caffeine and benzodiazepines. Careful observation of the patient is required during detoxification to identify withdrawal symptoms with potentially serious consequences.

The method of discontinuing the habituating drug is selected after considering the dosage of the agent, signs of tolerance, and the setting in which withdrawal will occur. For some patients who are on high doses of narcotics, barbiturates, and benzodiazepines, and who show signs of tolerance, the only safe method of drug discontinuation may be a gradual withdrawal. However, for the average patient using moderate amounts of these agents, abrupt withdrawal may be safely accomplished in the inpatient unit, where adequate precautions for the management of withdrawal symptoms are established.

The most typical signs and symptoms of withdrawal from opioids include sweating, yawning, tearing, a runny nose, tremors, muscle twitching, aching bones, muscle pain, irritability, pupil dilation, and an increased respiratory rate. These symptoms will occur during the first 24 hours and will be followed during the next two days by rapid heartbeat, hypertension, nausea, vomiting, insomnia, and abdominal cramps. As the process associated with detoxification subsides over a 5-to-10-day period, only symptomatic treatment will be required. However, specific treatment may be necessary, depending on the symptoms and their severity. The withdrawal symptoms will occur even with

246

those narcotics, such as codeine and pentazocine, that are generally considered safe and have minimal tendencies to produce habituation.

Barbiturate habituation frequently occurs in headache patients, since several of the prescription analgesics contain short-acting barbiturates. Withdrawal from these medications is frequently prolonged, and observation of the patient during the course of several weeks may be necessary. The typical signs and symptoms of barbiturate withdrawal include anxiety, insomnia, overactive reflexes, sweating, nausea, vomiting, rapid heartbeat, rapid breathing, and fever. Severe withdrawal symptoms from high doses of barbiturates may induce delirium and convulsive states, including grand mal epilepsy. Excessive amounts of caffeine, a common additive in both over-the-counter and prescription analgesics, produce withdrawal symptoms such as rebound vascular headaches, grogginess, malaise, runny nose, nausea, and depression.

The therapy program for the hospitalized patient is individualized, based on diagnosis and the patient's previous response to therapy. The medication used for pain relief for headaches may be a simple nonnarcotic analgesic, ergot, or a related drug, but strict limits in intake and total consumption should be emphasized. In addition, adjunctive prophylactic (preventive) therapy is also initiated for the headache problem, as well as for other physical and psychological signs and symptoms.

The pain from chronic tension-type headache is usually treated with simple nonnarcotic analgesics. Oxygen by mask is used as an adjunctive measure in treating the acute pain of cluster headaches.

Other medical therapies may be instituted if complicating medical problems exist. Prophylactic therapy is essentially required for all patients admitted to an inpatient unit. The choice of the agents is based on the initial evaluation and previous treatment responses.

Nearly all the patients admitted to our inpatient unit have complicated headache problems. Previous single-drug therapy may not have been adequate treatment for such problems, and several medications may be required for

247

headache prevention. For example, for patients with both migraine and tension-type headache, the use of propranolol in combination with a tricyclic antidepressant may be helpful.

Recognizing the increased risk of side effects from the combined use of multiple medications, initial observations, and management within the hospital environment facilitates prompt treatment if complications should arise. Alteration of medical therapy to avert side effects and adverse reactions is also possible.

The use of two medications in the prophylactic treatment of migraine or mixed headaches is best termed *copharmacy*. Copharmacy refers to medical treatment aimed at relieving certain well-defined target symptoms of migraine or mixed headache problems. This type of treatment has drawn criticism within the psychiatric community, particularly in the treatment of patients with coexisting depression and psychotic symptoms.

Sometimes, chronic pain, including headache, may be a manifestation of psychological problems. Accurate diagnosis by qualified psychologists and psychiatrists is essential if development of a long-term treatment program is necessary. The psychological manifestations of chronic headache somewhat resemble the characteristics of other chronic pain syndromes. Treatment for the chronic headache patient attempts to identify the specific components of suffering and pain behaviors. Encouraging "well behavior" is a vital aspect of this treatment. Patients are expected to wear street clothes and participate as a group in a variety of therapeutic and recreational programs.

Specific psychological intervention occurs on two levels. Group therapy sessions, such as assertiveness training, are conducted with a focus on problems common to headache patients. If indicated, individual psychological counseling is also initiated during the first few days of hospitalization and continued, as necessary, during and after hospitalization. Psychological tests are performed in accordance with the initial diagnosis of the physicians and psychologists. These tests may contribute valuable information and enhance both the initial treatment of the patient and long-term outpatient care.

Depression is often observed in headache patients. This may be manifested as a daily chronic tension-type headache or as a component of migraine. Anxiety is also a common aspect of a patient's pain behavior, whether or not that patient has specific pain complaints.

Biofeedback techniques, which are also part of the inpatient program, have proven to be useful in the treatment of migraine and tension-type headaches. For example, the migraine patient benefits from hand-warming techniques using finger temperature feedback. For patients with muscle contraction, mixed, and migraine headaches, feedback of electromyography potentials of the scalp and neck muscle is used. These techniques offer some benefit to approximately 70 percent of headache patients.

Intensive biofeedback treatment in the initial stages of therapy helps the patient to quickly integrate these skills. In order to further facilitate the patient's understanding of biofeedback training, a discussion group led by a biofeedback technician is provided. Outpatient reinforcement sessions may be coordinated with other aspects of treatment. Biofeedback, however, is only part of the therapy and should not be considered the single criterion for hospitalization.

Acupuncture is also encouraged during the hospital stay. Many patients find this to be a beneficial adjunctive therapy, and there is evidence in the headache literature that acupuncture can be helpful in migraine patients.

Physical and recreational therapy are also vital aspects of the inpatient program. The physical therapy department provides an optional exercise program for the inpatient and provides massage and diathermy as needed. A recreational therapy encourages the patients to participate in arts and crafts sessions as well as art therapy, stress management, relaxation exercises, and leisure planning. These techniques are useful for several reasons: they alter the pain behavior of the patient and provide alternative methods of coping with discomfort. Art therapy enables patients to gain a new perspective on their pain by transferring vague emotional images into more identifiable mental concepts and by viewing pain through inanimate objects. Guidance about use of leisure time enables patients to participate in planning for their eventual discharge.

Education of the headache patient also is essential to further the patient's understanding of the headache problem and to ensure a successful treatment program. Physicians, psychologists, pharmacists, and dietitians provide instruction. A discussion group, chaired by one of the staff physicians, highlights the general aspects of the headache treatment. A meeting with a staff pharmacist focuses on the actions of the specific medications, their side effects, drug interactions, and expected results. A class is held with a dietitian who discusses the tyramine-free diet, with special instruction for patients on MAO inhibitors. Menu planning for the headache patient is also described.

Furthermore, a weekly staff meeting is attended by representatives from each department—nursing, psychology, biofeedback, dietary, pharmacy, physical therapy, recreational therapy, social services, and utilization review. Each patient's diagnosis, therapy, and management are discussed. Other vital issues regarding the unit, such as patients' concerns about hospital regulations, are also reviewed at these meetings. In addition, interesting cases of hospitalized patients or cases that include a rare diagnosis are presented. On occasion, the case of a patient with an organic headache and with abnormal diagnostic studies will be presented, and X-rays or surgical reports will be discussed by the professional staff.

In summary, an inpatient unit may provide the last hope for many patients with intractable headache problems that have been unresponsive to therapy. Comprehensive evaluations beginning with carefully elicited patient histories are of utmost importance. Therapeutic measures can then be initiated that use an effective concept of inpatient headache treatment for those patients who have not succeeded in conventional outpatient therapy. This type of well-integrated, multidisciplinary approach has resulted in a 70 percent improvement in these patients following their discharge from the inpatient units.

250

33

COMMON QUESTIONS ABOUT HEADACHES

Here are some of the more common questions asked about headaches and their pain, together with the simplest and most direct answers I can provide.

What hurts during a headache?
Anything but the brain. The brain itself is insensitive to pain. You can cut it, poke it, freeze it, stick a needle into it, and it will not in itself hurt. What does hurt are such things as the blood vessels in the scalp, for example, when they become swollen or distended; the muscles of the face, the neck, and the scalp; or the protective covering around the brain (the meninges) when it becomes disturbed for any reason.

Do many people get headaches?
Almost everybody gets an occasional superficial headache, from poor posture, perhaps, from being in a stuffy room, or from a hangover. But what we're talking about in this book is the very severe and recurring kind of headache, the kind that forces you to stop what you're doing and take to your bed or to seek relief. I estimate that at least 37 million people in the United States suffer this kind of headache. At a very conservative estimate, that's about one in every eight persons in the country. Some experts in the field of headache would put the estimate at over 41 million.

Are all these people suffering from migraine headaches?
No, not at all. Migraine is a very severe and tormenting kind of headache, but not all headache sufferers really have migraine. Tension- type headache is actually more common than migraine, but when a patient's headache is severe and burdensome enough that he or she seeks the advice of a physician for the

headache, it is overwhelmingly migraine. Some studies estimate that as many as 13% of U.S. adults have migraine, and 2-3 million Americans have chronic migraine. Studies suggest that tension-type headache occurs in up to 78% of the population. Usually tension-type headaches do not negatively impact people's lives like migraine, however.

How many other kinds of headaches are there?
There are very severe headaches due to anxiety or depression, for example. There are headaches due to eyestrain, hunger, high blood pressure, low blood sugar, glaucoma, blood clots in the skull, brain tumors, painful facial tics, arthritis, neuralgia, meningitis, aneurysms, and so on.

What's the most common kind of headache?
The most common kind of headache is tension-type headache. The majority of the headache victims seen by a physician, however, are suffering from migraine. Most patients with tension-type headache do not seek medical advice for it— they take the occasional ibuprofen or acetaminophen and are fine. Once the patient suffers enough to miss school or work and ultimately speak to their healthcare provider about it, the headache is overwhelmingly likely to be migraine.

How can I tell if I've got a headache due to depression or anxiety?
The surest and swiftest way is to go to a doctor, preferably one who is interested in the treatment of headache.

What does the doctor want to know?
Tell the doctor where the pain is. In depression and anxiety headaches, you often find the pain as a pinched sense in the back of the neck at the base of the skull. Or frequently, it is a dull constant sensation that seems to go all around the head. We call this the "hatband effect."

- Tell the doctor how often you get the pain.
- The doctor will want to know at what time of day you get the pain. Patients with depression often get their headaches early in the morning or, alternatively, in the early evening before going to bed.
- The doctor will also want to know whether you find it difficult to sleep, and when. Patients with depression usually have trouble staying asleep and have frequent awakening. They awaken very early in the morning—4 or 5 o'clock—and can't go back to sleep. Patients with anxiety, on the other hand, have trouble falling asleep. They'll go to bed and toss and turn for hours.

How can I tell if I have a migraine headache?

The only way you can tell for sure is by going to a doctor who is interested in treatment of the headache. The doctor will want to know if you have the following signs of migraine:

- Often the pain of migraine is in the front of the head, and often but not always on one side or the other of the front of the head. (The term migraine is a French word that is derived from the Greek word, hemikrania, which means "half the head.")
- Do you get the pain only once or twice or perhaps three times a month? If the headache occurs more than 15 days per month, you may have chronic migraine.
- Do you get sick to your stomach and often vomit during the attack? (This is why migraine is so often called a "sick" headache. The majority of migraine patients have nausea, but the majority actually do not vomit.
- Do you "see things" a short while before the pain strikes? About 20 or 30 minutes before some, but not all, migraine attacks, the victim "sees" flashing lights or the sun rising sharply or stars exploding or other phenomena such as dots, people with halos or rainbows around them,

253

or even very grotesque images of humans or animals. Only 20 to 30 percent of migraine sufferers have warning symptoms. (Lewis Carroll, who had migraine, is believed to have taken some of the grotesqueries he saw before his migraine attacks and used them for some of the characters in his books *Alice in Wonderland* and *Alice Through the Looking Glass*.)

A few people will experience a change in other senses and sensations. They may get a funny taste in their mouths before the onset of migraine pain, or they may smell strange or repulsive odors. They may feel that their hands are getting cold. And some of those that suffer visual changes may find that some or all their vision is lost for a while.

Beyond all this, there is sometimes a change in mood. A certain number of migraine victims become highly euphoric before an onset of an attack; not only are they "high," so to speak, but they feel compelled to get a great deal of work done and, in fact, they get much more work done than in a comparable non-euphoric period. But after the migraine attack, after the pain has gone away, they feel very much let down from their "high."

Someone in the family who also has migraine is a most important factor in making a diagnosis of migraine. In fact, 80 percent of migraine sufferers have at least one first degree relative who also has migraine. This sibling or parent or child may have a very different set of symptoms and frequency of headache, however.

How do I know if I have a headache due to a brain tumor?
There's no way you can know other than by going to a doctor and having a series of tests. Some of the tests are quite simple and can be performed in the office. They will give some indications as to whether there is something significantly wrong, in a physical sense, with your brain or spinal cord or central nervous system. Other tests are more complex and must be performed in the

hospital. Between these various kinds of tests, a doctor can usually determine whether, in fact, you have a brain tumor.

What percentage of people actually have brain tumors?

The fact is that very few headache patients have brain tumors. I would put the figure at well under 0.5 percent. It is, of course, a useful precaution to be concerned about the possibilities of a tumor and to go to a doctor as soon as the suspicion arises. But that does not mean you should be worried over the inevitability of a brain tumor by the sudden onset of headache pain. I am surprised by the great number of patients who, even though they have a headache history lasting for 10 to 20 years, still worry needlessly about a brain tumor.

Is it true that a headache caused by a brain tumor is always more severe than, say, that caused by migraine?

No, this is not true. There is no way to tell whether a person has a brain tumor or not by the severity of the headache. Migraine pain can be just as severe as a brain tumor headache.

I've heard doctors use the term vascular headache. What is a vascular headache?

Vascular is simply the medical term for "vessel carrying the blood," that is, "blood vessel." A vascular headache, therefore, involves the blood vessels in the scalp or meninges (covering of the brain). What happens, in fact, is that these blood vessels swell and, as they become distended, cause pain. Migraine belongs to this category of headache. We have learned through research that, while there is indeed a vascular component to migraine, that there are changes that occur in the trigeminal nerve - specifically at a point in the brainstem called the trigeminal nucleus caudal - that incite a cascade of events, including the release of substances including CGRP that lead to the eventual pain and other symptoms of migraine. Generally speaking, the term "vascular headache" is not so widely used by headache specialists these days to describe migraine, but there is a vascular component.

Less common but more painful is another kind of vascular headache called a cluster headache (the pain comes in clusters, in two, three, four, or more headaches a day, each separated by many minutes or an hour or so of relief). A migraine headache, on the other hand, will sear on for 12 to 18 hours or more (and sometimes for two or more days) without relief.

The vascular headache is one of three rather broad classifications of headaches that those of us in the headache field have set up to describe headache pain and then to treat it.

What are the other two kinds of headache classification?
One headache classification is the tension-type headache. This term has replaced the older "muscle contraction headache" label. The tension-type headache is characterized by a tightening of the muscles in the neck, the head, or the face. As these muscles become very, very taut, they cause pain. The "hatband" pain of a tension-type headache is due to the tightening of the muscles all around the head.

The secondary headache is the other headache classification. This term describes a headache due to some organic problem in the body, whether it's a blood clot in the covering of the brain, glaucoma, high blood pressure, or any one of many other causes.

Is migraine more common in one sex than another?
Yes. Estimates vary, but most specialists in the field estimate that 60 to 80 percent of the migraine patients they see are women.

Can migraine occur at any age?

Yes, up to the middle years. It is rare that we see a new attack of migraine coming on a person who's over 45 or 55 years of age.

Most migraine attacks seem to come on first in the teenage years and then in the 20s. But I've had many patients who had their first migraine attack in their 30s. Migraine sometimes attacks children before their teens. There's even a special category of migraine relating to "motion sickness," which many children suffer. They get nauseated and want to vomit and then suffer headache pains. Many of us in the field believe that the biliousness and colic and young children and infants may be the early manifestations of migraine. There is no need to believe, though, that such headaches will necessarily be with them all through their young adulthood. On occasion, we see in the Headache Clinic a person with migraine who is so young that he or she can't even describe the pain. But the youngster suffers nausea and vomits and sometimes indicates that he or she is "seeing things."

You say that migraine does not often attack a person past his or her middle years, yet I've heard of people 50 or 60 years old, or older, who seem to be getting migraine. What about that?
I never say "never," I say "rarely." It is very rare for genuine migraine to begin in an older person for the first time. In fact, the migraine pain seems to go away, usually, after the middle years, although the visual signals, the aura, may continue for a long while.

When an older patient describes what appears to be a migraine headache attacking for the first time, the doctor would be wise to investigate it as a warning of another and more permanent vascular disorder becoming manifest.

Does migraine pain ever strike any place other than the head?
Yes. There is a form of migraine in which the pain strikes in the abdomen. It is called, quite naturally, abdominal migraine.

In this attack, the victim may get some of the usual signals of a migraine attack: the aura before his or her eyes, the nausea, and perhaps the vomiting, but when the pain comes, it comes to the abdomen. It is very intense and may last 12 to 18 hours, as long as migraine in the head might last. The pain also has the character of the migraine in the head; that is, it is throbbing, severe pain that, if it lasts long enough, may lose its pulsing nature and become constant. It is not unusual for a person with abdominal migraine to lose the pain in the abdomen after a number of years, only to see it turn up in the head in one of the more familiar forms of migraine.

A person who has abdominal migraine may encounter the same problem that the usual migraine patient suffers: the doctor can't find any reason for it. It is all the more mystifying, since it occurs in the abdominal region where we usually associate pain with organic causes. So, the patient is driven to distraction and desperation by this intense pain in his or her abdomen for which there is no explanation. It is not until or unless the pain moves to the head and the patient goes to a headache specialist and mentions the pain in the stomach area he or she has had all these years that the patient is likely to get an explanation for it.

You talk of different forms of migraine. How many kinds of migraine headache are there?
Some very thoughtful specialists in the headache field assign a migraine to every "cause"; that is, one due to changes in the hormonal balance, another due to the eating of foods with a chemical called tyramine, another due to repressed emotions, another due to certain chemicals that cause sensitivity (such as monosodium glutamate), even those due to a change in barometric pressure.

But all of us simply divide migraine headaches into two very broad categories: migraine with aura and migraine without aura. In migraine with aura, the patient gets the aura, the sense of nausea, and the throbbing pain. In migraine without aura, the aura may be missing but the pain is not. Most migraine victims

258

have migraine without aura. I'd say that only 20 to 30 percent of the migraine patients we see have migraine with aura.

There are some rare forms of migraine such as ophthalmoplegic migraine in which there is paralysis of the muscles controlling eye movement, and hemiplegic migraine in which there may be some temporary paralysis with the headache; there is a very rare form of migraine known as basilar-type migraine which has other troubling symptoms, including vertigo, hearing loss, difficulty speaking, ringing in the ears, and double vision in addition to the headache.

What happens to make the difference between migraine without aura and migraine with aura?
In all migraine headaches, as we've seen, there is a swelling (dilation) of the blood vessels in the scalp and covering of the brain.

It used to be thought that only in migraine with aura, the blood vessels constrict, or narrow, before they begin to swell, and that it was this constriction which lessens the blood supply to the brain and causes the victim to "see things." This is no longer thought to be the case, but that perhaps all migraine patients may experience aura, but that it is too faint to be noticed by the patient. Therefore, migraine with aura and migraine without aura actually may be much more similar in mechanism than was originally thought.

What cause the blood vessels to change size?
There are a number of chemical substances in and around the brain that seem to change before and during a migraine attack. We have identified at least five of them and there may be more. One important chemical is calcitonin gene-related peptide (CGRP). CGRP plays a very important role in vasodilation (opening of blood vessels). This peptide is the target of several new medications that serve to block the action of CGRP, thus inhibiting vasodilation.

259

As these substances change, so also does the size of the blood vessels. Another chemical called serotonin also can causes the blood vessels to constrict. Activation of the trigeminovascular system, due in part to the action of CGRP, leads to a cascade of events that causes the pain and other symptoms of migraine.

Is there anything else that happens to the blood vessels during a migraine attack?

Yes. Many of us now believe that the blood vessels become inflamed during a migraine attack. After all, simple swelling of the blood vessels would not account for the prolonged and acute pain of the migraine attack. You could, for example, get the blood vessels in your head to swell by taking a very long, very hot bath, but you would not get the pain of migraine.

This inflammation does not involve an infection (as would, say, a cut on your arm that becomes grievously inflamed), so we call it a "sterile" inflammation, and we now think this accounts for a good deal of the prolonged pain in migraine.

Is there anything that touches off the migraine attack?

Yes, we know of many things that might trigger an attack of migraine. The most familiar one, in women, is an influx of certain female hormones, most conspicuously estrogen. This takes place during the menstrual period and in those who take birth control pills and hormonal supplements.

But there are other triggers: hunger is one (perhaps because it lowers the blood sugar level); stress is another, repressed emotions are another. Indeed, there is a whole span of possible triggers from eating certain foods to experiencing a change in barometric pressure.

What we do not know is precisely why all these different triggers cause the migraine-sensitive chemicals in and around the brain to start changing, but

260

activation of the trigeminovascular system, as noted earlier, seems to an important step in the process of a migraine attack.

Why does oversleeping seem to trigger migraine attacks?
As we sleep, we build up levels of carbon dioxide (CO_2). This buildup will dilate the arteries around the head, and in turn trigger the pain. Also, to the extent that oversleeping interrupts a person's typical pattern of behaviors, this can trigger a migraine attack. One way to think of it is that "the migraine brain likes to have consistency." When that consistency is interrupted, a migraine attack can be triggered

I've heard there is a family factor in migraine. Is this true?
Yes, the family factor is at least partially true. We do see some patients who have no family history of migraine, but the number of cases in which there is a family factor is striking.

One piece of research focused on husband-and-wife combinations in which both partners had migraine. It showed that 91 percent of the parents of these patients had migraine and that 83 percent of the children of these couples also had migraine episodes. That seemed to be a powerful indication of migraine passing through three generations of a family. It is estimated that each child of a migraine patient has more than a 60 percent chance of having migraine. Again, the characteristics of the child's migraine may be quite different from that of the parent.

Doesn't that suggest that it's hereditary?
Yes, of course it does, but it doesn't fully explain why people without a family history of the ailment get migraine. Nor does it explain just what kind of hereditary pattern there is in migraine.

It may be that there is some inclination to migraine that is passed down from one generation to another, perhaps through some subtle enzyme effect. But

261

it may also be that there's a cultural inheritance of the migraine. In such a case, a child watches a parent with migraine and perhaps observes the special treatment that he or she gets from the rest of the family; then the child begins to imitate the parent's headache pattern to get that same special treatment. And before you know it, the child has a genuine migraine headache.

Is there a scientific basis for the belief that migraine is hereditary?
According to the genetic code theory, migraine is passed down from one generation to another through a gene, which makes a person susceptible to migraine when he or she is exposed to a condition that triggers the migraine. That might explain why migraine is touched off by hormonal changes in some people, by hunger in others, by stress in still others, or by certain kinds of food in yet others, and so on.

It might also explain why it strikes both men and women (whereas the hormonal trigger would suggest that women alone are susceptible), and why it strikes people of all ages—infants as well as young women reaching puberty. (The gene not only determines that a certain kind of action takes place, but also when it takes place. The time factor may vary from person to person.) To date, genetic mutations have been identified in one rather rare type of migraine, familial hemiplegic migraine. This is certainly a very important step toward our having a better understanding of the genetic basis of migraine. But, although this is a very attractive field of research, it holds no early likelihood of a miracle cure for migraine—if such a cure should ever exist.

Is there a particular kind of person who gets migraine?
Again yes—a qualified yes. Many migraine patients are perfectionists in most of the things they do. They are often described as having a "Type A" personality. They tend to be intelligent and to be doers and achievers. However, the psychological makeup of migraine sufferers tends to be similar to that of non-

migraine sufferers, pointing to a physical rather than a psychological basis for migraine.

Is a headache in itself a disease, one that you can find a miracle cure for?
No. A headache is merely a symptom of something else that's wrong in the body or psyche. The "something wrong" may be very direct, such as a blood clot in the covering of the brain (meninges). Or perhaps it's due to high blood pressure or eye problems or any of several other problems.

Or the "something wrong" may be in the victim's environment; for example, too much carbon monoxide being inhaled in a stuffy garage, drinking too much liquor, or reacting to something disturbing in the individual's lifestyle—a wrong direction, perhaps, or a wrong pace.

The importance of headache is great, in any case. For it is the only medical symptom to which an entire medical association is devoted—the American Headache Society. There is also an international medical association devoted to headache—the International Headache Society.

Because it is a symptom, and, for that matter, a symptom of any number of medical conditions, there is no single cure for a headache, nor is there likely to be a miracle cure soon.

How does this relate to migraine?
Migraines are perhaps the most difficult of headaches to attack. We can reduce them in severity and in frequency, but we do not often succeed in ending them altogether. What we can do is put the patient in control of his or her headaches instead of having the headaches in control of the patient.

Are there any signs common to migraine other than the aura, the nausea, and the headache pain?
As the attack progresses, the migraine victim usually becomes very sensitive to light and to sound; I might say hypersensitive. Light and sound of almost any

263

kind seem to contribute enormously to the victim's pain. There can also be a sense of coldness in the hands and sometimes in the feet.

Finally, and most importantly, the pain often seems to concentrate on one side of the head or the other, often behind one of the eyes. In migraine with aura, it tends to strike always on the same side of the head. In migraine without aura, the pain may strike one side of the head in one headache, and then strike the other side in the next headache. Occasionally the headache may occur on both sides of the head or in the entire head.

How often are the headaches concentrated on one side?
In well over 70 percent of the cases.

What happens in the other cases?
The indication is that the pain will move across the forehead from one side to the other.

Isn't it possible to mistake migraine for something else?
Because the pain is located in the face and forehead, there's an inclination by some to mistake it for a sinus infection. We commonly see migraine headaches misdiagnosed and treated as sinus headaches, in fact it is one of the most common misdiagnoses made by primary care physicians. But if the full migraine hits—the aura, the pain, the nausea, the sensitivity to light and sound, the coldness of the extremities—there is little likelihood it will be mistaken, by a qualified observer, for anything else.

How does pregnancy affect migraine?
Often, by the second or third month of pregnancy, the migraine attacks will disappear until after the birth of the child. Note that I say "often." The pregnancy relief takes place in the clear majority of cases, but not in every case.

Why should the migraine disappear during pregnancy?

Because the hormonal balance in the woman changes during pregnancy. There is a lessening of the variability of certain female hormones. The variability of estrogen that occurs during a menstrual cycle, most probably when the levels of estrogen drop, is often a trigger of migraine. Without this variability, migraines often improve.

What can be done for a woman suffering a migraine attack during pregnancy?

Fortunately, most women cease getting migraines by the third month of pregnancy. There is an FDA warning against the use of the triptans during pregnancy. However, sumatriptan has been studied extensively in pregnant patients, and the result to date has been that there is no greater incidence of miscarriage or birth defects recorded above those in the general population. Therefore, we tend to allow pregnant patients to take sumatriptan, if necessary, as long as it is cleared by their OB/GYN. We always make sure the patient understands that the FDA warning exists, and that the lack of an observed increased incidence of miscarriage and birth defects does not mean that such an increased risk does not exist. Otherwise acetaminophen is recommended.

Does it follow, then, that an increase in levels of the female hormones may contribute to migraine?

The answer is—sometimes. That is to say, one-third of women who start birth control pills will see an increase in pain and frequency, but one-third of them may see a decrease, while another one-third may not see any change whatsoever. It seems that the most predictable trigger from estrogen is the change in estrogen concentration in the body, specifically the rapid decrease in levels. Even this is not always predictable, however.

Now isn't the reverse true—that a decrease in female hormones during menopause will decrease migraine?

Yes, that is true—once menopause has completed and there are no longer fluctuations in estrogen levels in the body. We usually find that migraine decreases or altogether disappears after menopause. However, there are some women who take female hormones during menopause, usually to reduce some of the menopausal symptoms. This, of course, tends to nullify the impact of menopause and thus to prolong or increase the severity and frequency of migraine pain.

In all of this, you must remember, we are speaking of migraine that is triggered by hormonal changes. There are a good many other factors, such as consuming certain foods, that may trigger a migraine attack.

What are some of the foods that may trigger a migraine attack?

Freshly baked bread, port, cheese (except for cottage cheese), herring, yogurt, navy beans, lima beans, most citrus fruits, vinegar (except white vinegar), onions, nuts, and chocolates.

These foods trigger migraine only in certain migraine-prone individuals, not in the normal headache-free individual. I very strongly urge my migraine patients to avoid eating these foods.

Why do migraine victims have to skip these foods?

Skipping these foods simply helps reduce the frequency and intensity of migraine attacks. The foods mentioned above all contain a chemical agent, tyramine, which is known to set into motion certain circulatory and hormonal changes in the body. The exception to this is chocolate, which doesn't contain actual tyramine, but a chemical agent that is a very close relative to it, phenethylamine, which has much the same effect on migraine as tyramine.

Is there anything a migraine victim must skip in the way of drinking?

Oh, yes. The migraine victim must avoid beer, red wine, bourbon, gin, vodka, in general, anything that is fermented.

Is there anything the migraine sufferer can drink?
Yes. We've found that rose wine, white wine (except Sauternes), brandy, cordials, Scotch, and rum will not cause a tyramine reaction in migraine patients. However, even the acceptable alcoholic beverages must never be taken in excess by the migraine patient.

Are all migraine patients susceptible to tyramine?
No, we find that only about 50 percent of them have a sensitivity to tyramine. But because we don't know which 50 percent when we start treatment, we recommend to all our migraine patients that they go on a tyramine-free diet. It just gives us an extra edge in trying to curb the pain and incidence of migraine.

How do you go about treating a migraine patient?
In general, doctors specializing in treating the headache follow a two-part program. First, they try to attack the pain of migraine, to reduce it in severity and to reduce the frequency of the attacks. This is usually accomplished by prescribing one of a variety of medicines that seem to have an impact on migraine pain. If one doesn't work, the doctor will then go on to try another until he or she finds one that will work in the right dosage.

Second, they try to find the underlying cause of the migraine pain (or, for that matter, of any headache pain). If they can find it, they then try to eliminate it.

It's usually easier to reduce the pain of migraine than to find and eliminate its underlying cause because the causes are sometimes quite subtle. Indeed, sometimes they are beyond the conscious reach of the patient. Many patients will need prophylactic therapy with a drug such as propranolol.

But reducing the pain and frequency of the attacks is, in my view, a useful achievement. For migraine pain often comes close to destroying the personality, even the life, of its victim. Often, he or she finds it impossible to accomplish even the minimum functions of day-to-day living because the pain is so constant and intense. By greatly decreasing the pain, we may be able to return the patient to a useful and fulfilling life—to one that has more gratifications than frustrations.

How do you go about attacking the pain of migraine?
There are two general approaches to it: one is called abortive therapy, the other is called prophylactic (preventive) therapy.

What is abortive migraine therapy?
Abort means "to interrupt." We simply interrupt the headache after it signals that is about to begin. (One signal in migraine with aura is, of course, the aura—the sense of seeing things—that takes place 20 or 30 minutes before the actual pain of migraine.) By giving the patient a carefully prescribed medicine at the first signal of the onset of the migraine, we are usually able to abort the headache.

What medicines are the most effective in abortive therapy?
In the 1970s, the scientists at Glaxo in the United Kingdom began investigation trying to identify the serotonin receptor type responsible for the beneficial effect of serotonin. The research team, led by Patrick P.A. Humphrey, discovered the serotonin receptor type 5-HT1B, which is mainly found in cranial rather than peripheral blood vessels. This discovery enabled them to design novel agonists which specifically stimulated these receptors to produce selective vasoconstriction of the cranial vessels, which can become distended and inflamed. In 1988, the prototypical triptan, sumatriptan, was administered parenterally; it demonstrated efficacy and was well tolerated in most patients. In

the U.S., it became available in 1992 after publication of the results of two parallel-group trials in the acute treatment of migraine. Originally available only for subcutaneous administration, other forms were eventually approved, including oral, intranasal, and subcutaneous.

At Merck's Neuroscience Center in the U.K., Richard Hargreaves and his team discovered the triptan rizatriptan. Other triptans followed, including zolmitriptan and eleptriptan. The 1990s have been called the decade of the "triptan wars".

The newest classification of headache, an addition called chronic migraine, has expanded our nomenclature. Chronic migraine is defined as migraine headache occurring on 15 or more days per month for more than three months.

Are these drugs helpful for all migraine headaches?

At one time it was thought that these drugs could be used effectively only in migraine with aura because that kind of migraine provided a signal (in the aura) that allowed the patient to consume the drug and offset the pain before the pain totally overwhelmed the victim. The theory was that once the pain gained momentum, it could not be checked. Now, after years of research and practice, we know that ergotamine tartrate and its compounds can help many of the migraine victims who have common, not classic migraine (the migraine that strikes without the warning of the aura). It will not help them all, but it will help most them. All they have to do is take the medicine at the first hint of pain and the ergotamine tartrate will abort the pain. Usually, it will be about 15 or 20 minutes before the medicine becomes effective.

Can everyone use triptans?

No triptans should be used by patients with certain kinds of cardiac (heart) conditions. As discussed earlier, there is an FDA warning against the use of triptans during pregnancy (presumably the migraine headaches will have dwindled anyway). A thoughtful discussion should be undertaken with the headache physician, the OB/GYN, and the patient prior to the use of a triptan during pregnancy. Moreover, triptans should not be used on a daily basis because a rebound reaction can occur causing daily headaches.

When do you consider using abortive therapy?
My own tendency is to use abortive therapy when the migraine attacks one to two times a month. In that way, we don't have to keep the patient taking medicine every day to ward off once-a-month migraine pain.

What, then, is preventive, or prophylactic therapy?
You've seen how, in abortive therapy, we try to interrupt the headache once it has gotten started. In preventive therapy, we try to keep the headache from even getting started. This is sometimes called prophylaxis, which is medical term for preventive therapy.

When is it used?
Usually, we use preventive therapy in patients who are having two or more migraine attacks a month, but this largely depends on the disability each attack causes, and how effective abortive therapy has been for the patient. Ultimately, the decision must be because I have determined with the patient that it is justifiable to have her on a daily regime of medicine to keep the headaches from having a chance to get started.

What medicines are used in preventive therapy?
There are several medicines which we prescribe to prevent the headaches from getting started. Propranolol (Inderal), a beta blocker, is one. These beta blockers are used to treat heart conditions primarily, and they were discovered, quite by accident, to also help prevent migraines. The treatment of choice for long-term prophylaxis is propranolol LA, which can be taken as a once-a-day dose.

Tricyclic antidepressants (such as amitriptyline, nortriptyline, and protriptyline) are prescribed to prevent the frequency and severity of migraine. In addition to tricyclic antidepressants, the serotonin-norepinephrine reuptake inhibitor (SNRI) venlafaxine (Effexor) can be effective in preventing migraine.

We also prescribe antiepileptic medications to prevent migraine. Topiramate (Topamax) and Sodium Valproate (Depakote) are both FDA-approved for the prevention of migraine.

Another useful class of medicines is the "nonsteroidal anti-inflammatories," such as ibuprofen (Motrin). There are certain drugs in this class that can be extremely useful in preventing migraine attacks. These are particularly helpful during women's menses. The side effects mainly involve an occasional feeling of sickness to the stomach.

An older, mild medicine, with few side effects, is particularly useful in children: cyproheptadine (Periactin). A further class of medicines being used is the calcium channel blockers, such as verapamil (Isoptin and Calan). Like the beta blockers (Inderal), these are primarily heart and blood pressure medicines, but they can be extremely useful in preventing migraine attacks.

Onabotulinum toxin A (BOTOX) is effective at reducing the frequency and severity of chronic migraine and is FDA-approved for this purpose.

Are there stronger medicines than those previously listed for preventing migraines?

Yes. There is the class of medicines called the monoamine oxidase (MAO) inhibitors. These can be very useful in patients who have not done well with the usual prophylactic medications. Because of the possible side effects, the patient is usually hospitalized in our inpatient headache unit when we begin this treatment.

Does a patient taking the MAO inhibitors need to practice any special precautions, and are there side effects?

Yes. Patients who are taking the drug must be very careful about their diets. They cannot eat any of the tyramine-containing foods mentioned earlier, plus certain other foods, such as chicken livers or pods of broad beans, for fear of bringing about a severe transient blood pressure problem. Similarly, they should not take other medicines without consulting their doctors (and I include such "cold remedies" as Sudafed (pseudoephedrine), and nose drops in this category). All alcoholic beverages are forbidden. While on an MAO inhibitor, such patients cannot take narcotics such as meperidine (Demerol), which are sometimes prescribed simply for their pain-killing properties. The reason is that these drugs in combination may cause a low blood pressure crisis. Patients on MAO inhibitors should be off the drug for at least two weeks before they have any major surgery involving anesthetics.

Are there any other drugs for the treatment of headache?
Yes. One is called clonidine (Catapres), an alpha blocker. It reduces the response of the blood vessels to substances that cause both vasodilation and vasoconstriction. As in the case of propranolol, clonidine cannot be discontinued abruptly but must be decreased over a few days and then stopped. It has not been proven to be more effective than propranolol.

What about good old aspirin? Doesn't that have any use in trying to combat headache?
Aspirin is perfectly acceptable for trying to mute the pain of the occasional headache. But is has very little impact on the deep and persistent pain of migraine or, for that matter, on other chronic and recurring headaches.

As a rule of thumb, two aspirin tablets provide the maximum possible effect that aspirin can have for a period of three or four hours. There is no need to take more than that in the three-to four-hour period. If you need to take more, then you know that aspirin will not do much to overcome your headache. And perhaps that is the best signal that you'd better go see a doctor if you want relief from headache pain.

What is chronic migraine?

For almost all the people having migraines, the extreme disruptions of the disease are intermittent and hopefully infrequent. In chronic migraine, it has transformed from a once- or twice-monthly disorder to a chronic disease capable of interfering and disrupting virtually every part of a person's life. It is characterized by repeated attacks of migraine occurring unpredictably, often for days on end, and occurring for many decades of a person's life. The diagnosis of chronic migraine is made when the person has 15 or more headache days per month for more than three months.

Migraine defines an individual's threshold for headaches. Migraineurs are more likely to develop headache as a symptom of a brain tumor or other secondary headache causes. Furthermore, the headache they subsequently develop is often similar to their original migraines, only more frequent and severe. Therefore, an individual with a progression or transformation of these attacks should be reevaluated to assure that they have not developed a secondary headache.

Is there any chance that aspirin might be damaging?

In small quantities, it is not damaging. But people with very severe headaches rarely stop at small quantities. They are much more inclined to gulp down more and more aspirin or aspirin-like compounds in an effort to quell the pain of any one headache, even though it does little good.

Just let it be said that an excessive amount of aspirin or similar compounds can cause kidney damage, chronic ulcer, and other stomach problems. Excessive aspirin intake causes a loss of blood from the intestinal tract and thus may cause chronic anemia. It may also cause some deviations from an otherwise normal pattern in neurological examinations.

All this is uncommon, but it is to be considered seriously by anybody who is consuming a great deal of aspirin.

What is the story regarding caffeine?

Caffeine, contained in coffee, tea, colas, chocolate, and so on, is a powerful drug that is actually a double-edged sword. It will help the pain of a headache, usually because of its blood-vessel-constricting properties, and is often found in combination with aspirin or butalbital. However, excessive caffeine use (more than the equivalent of three cups of coffee per day) will lead to further headaches. Moreover, one then becomes trapped in a cycle of needing the caffeine for the headache that was created by the caffeine in the first place.

How about cold packs?

These will help for most types of headache; they will even help the severe pain of migraine.

Is there any way of treating headaches without the use of drugs?

Yes. Adjunctive treatments, including biofeedback, acupuncture, physical therapy, and massage therapy, can be helpful in treating headaches.

What is biofeedback?

Bio is the Greek prefix meaning "life," as in the word biological. Feedback is a term for receiving information, in this case, on current behavior, which can be used to influence or modify future behavior. The word biofeedback is used to mean the process by which a patient is given instant information, on an ongoing and immediate basis, about mind and body events through the use of electronic instrumentation.

Biofeedback is a method which teaches patients to control certain functions of both their involuntary autonomic nervous system, such as heart rate and blood pressure, and their voluntary central nervous system, such as muscle tension.

In short, biofeedback is a tool used to teach patients to self-regulate specific biological functions.

Is biofeedback a psychological treatment?
Biofeedback is not a psychological, but rather a psychophysiological approach. It is physiological in the sense that it can be observed and measured. The "psycho" prefix means that is determined by the will of the patient.

Has biofeedback been proved effective scientifically?
Yes, there is considerable evidence from randomized clinical trials that supports the efficacy of biofeedback to treat migraine and tension-type headache, with estimates of improvement in headache of between 35 percent and 60 percent.

But how can you teach people to control things that happen automatically in the body?
This is done by a process called operant conditioning. Very sophisticated electronic equipment is used in the process. Instruments which monitor such functions as those mentioned before (heart rate, hand temperature, muscle tension, and so forth) are used to "feedback" to patients information which they could not be aware of on their own. For example, a person normally would not realize how often the temperature in his or her hand varies, let alone to what extent. With biofeedback instrumentation, we can monitor a patient's bodily functions and feed them back to the individual immediately as changes take place. Through this process—called operant conditioning—the patient can learn to control these functions.

For what kind of disorders is biofeedback used?

Biofeedback has been accepted as a viable therapeutic tool in the treatment of many disorders, including high blood pressure, Raynaud's disease, muscle spasm, chronic anxiety, neuromuscular reeducation, epilepsy, insomnia, asthma, and various other stress-related conditions. In this context, "stress-related" does not mean that the condition is caused by stress, but rather that stress can trigger the symptoms of the condition.

How successful is biofeedback in teaching patients to control headaches?
There have been many studies in recent years testing the efficacy of biofeedback training in the treatment of headaches. These studies have shown biofeedback to be a highly effective tool in the treatment of both migraine and tension-type headaches.

A four-year retrospective study done at the Diamond Headache Clinic and published in the January 1984 issue of *Headache*, the journal of the American Association for the Study of Headache, reports that of 693 patients, 83 percent reported an overall improvement due to biofeedback training. Of these patients, 40 percent had decreased their medication intake, and 18 percent had completely eliminated medication.

Since that original research, considerably more evidence from randomized clinical trials have emerged that supports the efficacy of biofeedback to treat migraine and tension-type headache, with estimates of improvement in headache of between 35 percent and 60 percent.

Does it take a long time to learn?
Biofeedback is a process that demands a certain amount of training. For most headache patients, the actual time of training with instruments can be as little as 10 sessions that are regularly attended on a once- or twice-a-week basis along with daily home practice. However, you must remember that the goal of biofeedback is to give the patient a tool with which he or she can retrain specific

physiological responses of the nervous system. Many of these responses are automatic. This retraining is done through operant conditioning, a learning process, and thus continued practice is necessary even after the initial series of sessions is completed.

Patients must practice on their own, under all kinds of conditions, what they have learned during the sessions. A number of follow-up sessions are also required, at longer and less regular intervals than the original series, to reinforce the learning process. However, many patients report a beneficial change in the frequency, severity, and duration of their headaches even during the initial ten sessions.

What kind of instruments are used?

In working with headache patients, the two types of instruments that are most often employed are the electronic thermometer, which is used for temperature training, and the electromyography (EMG), a device which measures muscle tension.

Does it hurt?

No, not at all. The instruments are used only to measure certain physiological events occurring in the body that the patient would not normally be aware of (such as hand temperature and muscle tension), and to feed that information back to the patient. Patients are attached to the instruments by way of topically placed sensors. In the case of temperature training, the sensor is a thermistor which is attached to the middle or index finger of the patient with tape. It merely measures the changes in finger temperature as they happen. In the case of electromyography (EMG) training, the sensors are attached to the patient with an adhesive strip that is placed on any of several areas which are often found to be tense in headache patients (such as the forehead, neck, shoulders, or jaw). The sensors monitor changes in muscle tension as they occur in these muscle groups.

What does a patient need to learn?

Headaches are best controlled when the patient has a combination of temperature and EMG training. Temperature training consists of learning to warm one's hands. When patients learn hand-warming, they are actually learning to direct more blood into their hands. Since the pain of the migraine headache is the result of an over dilation of blood vessels in the head, this "redirecting" of the blood can prevent this condition. The result is a reduction in the severity, duration, and/or frequency of the headaches.

Electromyograph training is a method for achieving muscle relaxation. The patient learns to differentiate muscle tension from muscle relaxation, to recognize when muscle tension begins to increase, and when and how to deeply relax those muscles that affect headache activity.

Patients are also taught the relaxation process by means of a number of relaxation techniques including autogenics, progressive relaxation, imagery, and breathing exercises. Diaphragmatic breathing is also taught.

Are you saying that I can get rid of my headaches by just learning to relax?

In a sense, yes, but the process is much more complicated. It is true that biofeedback is taught in a quiet, dimly lit room with the patient seated in a comfortable chair to enhance the proper physiological responses. However, the long-term goal of biofeedback training is to have patients, through continued practice, learn to do the tasks of hand-warming and muscle relaxation in real-life situations. This process, called generalization, is accomplished by way of behavior modification aids to help patients to bring what they have learned in training into use in everyday life. When the generalization process is accomplished, patients can readily prevent or abort headaches through self-regulation.

Which patients profit from biofeedback training?

278

Many different types of people can benefit from biofeedback. The most important components of successful biofeedback training are patient motivation, the ability to concentrate and learn to relax, and a willingness to become an active participant in the treatment.

Research has shown that young people are often particularly quick to learn biofeedback methods, but older patients certainly learn and benefit from it, too. However, biofeedback training is by no means the answer for all illnesses or all patients. It is critical that the assessment as to the appropriateness of biofeedback referral be made by a physician.

You mentioned that migraine is a form of vascular headache. What about cluster headache, the other form of vascular headache?

The cluster headache is a very severe form of headache. It occurs predominantly in men, and it involves a deep, burning pain within the head. Some cluster victims will literally beat their heads against the wall to escape the pain. I had one patient, a young man, who pleaded with his father to knock him out so that he would no longer suffer the pain. Some victims become so distracted by the pain that they consider suicide. It is so severe that we have a rule in our clinic that, although most of our appointments are booked several weeks in advance, we take a cluster victim immediately.

Why is it called a cluster headache?

Because it does not come on and last for 12 to 18 hours or two to three days, as does the migraine headache. Instead, it lasts for 30 minutes to two hours, then goes away for a while, then resumes and lasts another 30 minutes to two hours. It may come two or three or four or more times a day—in clusters.

Is this the only difference between it and migraine?

No. Migraine, as we've seen, is very unlikely to come every day. The cluster headache appears daily—when in season.

For again, unlike migraine, it is not a year-round torment. The cluster will strike its victim for a few weeks, perhaps for as many as two or three months. Then it goes away, thus encouraging the victim to think he or she is free of its torture, only to come back a few months later as intensely as ever. Some doctors have traced its seasons to spring and autumn, leading, or misleading them to associate it with the business tensions of these seasons (income tax and annual reports in the spring; new product sales and inventory buildup in autumn). Or they have come to associate it with allergies, which sometimes become active in the spring or fall. Actually, the seasons of the cluster headache may be somewhat individual and personal, striking when the particular victim is susceptible rather than on any scale of nature.

Do women ever get cluster headaches?
Yes, they do. We find that about one woman reports a cluster headache for every five men.

Are there any bodily changes connected with cluster headaches?
If you're thinking about a connection with the female menstrual period, as in migraine, no, there appears to be no connection between that and cluster headaches in women. We have found, however, that there is an increased incidence in peptic ulcers among both male and female cluster headache victims.

What about the appearance of patients with cluster?
Cluster victims tend to have a rugged appearance, a square jaw, somewhat thick facial skin, and a roughened appearance of the skin around the cheeks. The latter is called peau d'orange, meaning that the skin has some of the character of the skin of an orange. The forehead is also often furrowed, the lower lip is well chiseled, and the chin may even have a cleft.

Do women also turn up with the cluster appearance if they are victims of this kind of headache?

Yes, to the extent that it holds true for cluster victims in general, it also holds true for women.

Is there is a "cluster" personality?

Patients with cluster headaches do tend to be somewhat aggressive, hard-driving, and successful. The relationship between these personality traits and the cluster headaches is not clear.

How do the headaches develop?

They come on quite swiftly, often reaching full force within 5 or 10 minutes after the first signal of pain.

Do they come at any particular time of the day or night?

They can come at any time. But we do find an unusual number of the first cluster headaches coming during the night and waking the victim out of a sound sleep. Subsequently, clusters may follow a daytime pattern.

Is there any common characteristic in cluster headaches other than the pain?

Yes. The cluster headache comes on one side of the head, like the migraine. Usually, the cluster victim will find the eye on that side of the head watering during the headache. The nostril on that side of the head will likely become runny. And the skin on that side of the face will appear somewhat flushed.

Is there anything the patients themselves can do about it?

Virtually nothing. The thing most cluster victims do instinctively is to get up and start pacing agitatedly (where most migraine victims, as you'll recall, instinctively go to bed and try to sleep the pain away).

What can be done about cluster headaches?

There are many successful therapies for cluster headaches, both abortive and preventive. To stop the attack once it comes, oxygen and or sumatriptan are often used. Sumatriptan needs to get into the bloodstream quickly, so we use either a nasal spray or we may teach the patients to give themselves a sumatriptan injection. The patients keep oxygen at home and put on an oxygen mask as soon as the pain begins. This will often stop the headache. A short course of steroids can be very helpful but should be limited only to one or two weeks.

How about medicines to prevent clusters?

There are many useful drugs for this purpose. Certain steroids, helpful in treating arthritis, are very beneficial. Truthfully, though, the reason these drugs work well on cluster headaches is still obscure, but whatever the reason, they do work. Other very useful medications include lithium and the calcium channel blockers that were mentioned for migraines, such as verapamil (Calan and Isoptin). The anti-inflammatories, particularly indomethacin, also have some effect in treating clusters.

Is biofeedback also helpful in controlling cluster headaches?

Although research has not shown biofeedback to be of help in aborting or preventing cluster headaches, both muscle relaxation and diaphragmatic breathing are often of great help in pain management in general.

Is there any way to treat cluster headaches without drugs?

Yes, although not through biofeedback, as in migraine treatment. The cluster treatment is called histamine desensitization. In a strict sense, it does use a drug—histamine, a chemical found in the body—but the drug is not used for normal consumption to attack the headache pain the way other drugs are used.

Rather, it is used to fortify the patient against the impact of a change in the histamine level in his or her body.

Histamine is implicated by some but not by all headache specialists in the onset of cluster. Most people think of histamine as being a chemical agent that's a villain in many illnesses. It's the chemical agent that sometimes causes a stuffy nose during a cold or during the hay fever season. That's why people take antihistamines to combat the stuffy-nose feeling. Histamine is a substance that helps the body fight infection and injury. But it's been found to be anything but a protector by those researchers who are convinced that it has a profoundly important influence on cluster headache; that, indeed, it inspires the headache in those persons sensitive to it. The idea therefore, is to desensitize the cluster victim and to use histamine to do it.

How is this done?
The patient is admitted to our inpatient headache unit for 10 to 12 days. Each day, a small amount of histamine solution is dripped into the patient's veins, and the amount is gradually increased.

Does this method of treatment have any drawbacks?
One of the drawbacks, of course, is that by giving just a little too much histamine on any one day, you might ignite precisely the kind of headache that the treatment is supposed to help prevent. Some specialists in headache are not as enthusiastic as others about histamine desensitization. For our part, we find that it works in some cases and that it doesn't quite work in others—precisely like many of the other treatments in medicine.

You've said a lot about the vascular kind of headache. Now would you explain something about another category of headache that I might have?
By far the most common form of headache is the tension-type headache. Most people with tension-type headache will not seek medical treatment for it,

however, they will successfully treat it at home with the occasional ibuprofen or acetaminophen and a little bit of exercise or stretching.

Does one sex get this kind of headache more than the other?
Not necessarily.

Is there a family factor in these headaches?
Not really. Occasionally you'll see a child who might have learned the headache pattern from a parent and tends to imitate it. But that is not a genuinely important factor in overall consideration of the headache as a scientific phenomenon, although it may be important as a personal and individual one, particularly in treating the headache.

What cause the muscles to contract and tighten up?
There is a change in the chemicals in and around the brain, but these are not precisely the same chemicals that change in migraine.

Do depression and anxiety have any signals in common?
Yes, in both cases there is a pronounced sleep disturbance. Anxiety patients have trouble falling asleep, while depression victims have trouble staying asleep—they wake up in the wee hours of the morning and can't get back to sleep. In addition, people can have anxiety as part of their depression symptoms.

Are there any characteristics that suggest a headache is triggered by anxiety or depression?
Yes. Let's take depression patients for example:
- They are likely to tell you that they had the headaches all their lives. They haven't, it simply seems that long because they have been in the depression so long.

284

- The headaches come very often but seem to increase on weekends, holidays, and vacations.

- The pain does not respond to aspirin and other over-the-counter preparations.

- The pain seems greater in the early morning and again in the evening. That's natural because depression victims wake up early in the morning with their problem—the hours from 4 to 8 o'clock in the morning are those of the greatest silent personal and family crises. Victims fight through, in their minds, their work-related or family problems. Similarly, with the evening headaches, the confrontation of family problems arises between 4 and 8 o'clock at night after the victim has escaped them for most of the day.

Why should the headaches increase on weekends or holidays?

If the cause of the depression is some situation within the family, this kind of pattern may arise, particularly in a patient who works during the week.

At work, the patient is freed from contact with these problems and gets some relief from them. But on weekends and holidays, the patient knows he is going to face these problems for long stretches when he must appear comfortable and relaxed. In effect, the patient may feel he has to repress resentment against somebody he is expected to love and respect, and so he converts this conflict through a depression into a headache.

Also, oversleeping, or missing a meal, both of which can alter blood sugar levels, can precipitate a headache. Furthermore, a person who consumes excessive amounts of caffeine at work and less during the weekend may get a headache because of caffeine withdrawal.

Does depression cause any other symptoms?

Yes, very many. We find that about three out of four patients complain of problems involving the stomach or gastrointestinal tract; they complain of

285

constipation, losing weight, or loss of appetite. We find that about three out of five complain of some sexual problem—a decreased libido, for example. Other complaints range from palpitations to weakness and fatigue to changes in urination patterns.

On a less physical, more psychic level, a great many—91 percent— complain of a loss of concentration. Others—71 percent—say they have a poorer memory. About 75 percent say they've lost their drive and ambition, and the same percentage say they feel considerably less decisive. Generally, a cook may find that she can't follow a simple recipe, or a practiced bridge player may find that she is making consistent blunders when she is in a depression.

I've said that this kind of depression is considerably more severe than the everyday temporary sensation of "feeling blue." But depression victims do complain of feeling sad—some 90 percent of them report this emotional disturbance, and 80 percent report bursting into tears. But the feeling blue sensation is only a part of the overall picture of depression; it does not constitute the total picture of depression as we are discussing it here.

Also, we often find that the victim of depression is markedly introverted and tends to dwell on his or her illnesses. That individual also comments on his or her mistakes in a self-deprecating manner.

And when the victim tries to explain—to himself or even to the doctor—why he should feel this way, that person attributes it to some specific event in the past (perhaps an auto accident) rather than the job or family or other present conflict which is likely to have precipitated it.

But aren't there identifiable incidents which might throw a person into a depression, such as the loss of a loved one?
I think you're talking about grief rather than depression. Grief is a perfectly natural response to the loss of a loved one. It is accepted as normal when it does not last for an extended period (i.e., years) and when it does not overshadow the whole existence of the patient for that time. If it lasts too long, it may, to be sure,

settle into a prolonged and clinical depression in which headache is almost a daily occurrence. That person should be aware of this; certainly, other members of the family must observe it. It is imperative to prevent the sense of grief from overflowing into a prolonged experience of deep depression. But in all candor, I must confess that grief as a cause of depression is not common, nor are auto or other accidents. The most familiar causes of depression are rooted elsewhere in family relationships or in job conflicts.

How do you go about treating a headache triggered by depression?
This is one of those instances where you attack the pain by attacking the depression. To be sure, we don't get at the cause of depression right away—not in the first visit, anyway. But we can relieve the depression by chemical means, and by doing that, we can start to relieve the headache pain. I always encourage the patient to engage in psychotherapy, as this will have a favorable impact not only on the depression, but the headache as well.

What are the chemical means?
You've seen what I've said about the decrease of the chemical agents called catecholamines in the brain when a person is in a depression and about selecting medicines which preserve or increase them.

One group of drugs which help preserve them is called the tricyclic antidepressants: amitriptyline, protriptyline, and nortriptyline. Others are imipramine (Tofranil), desipramine (Norpramin), and doxepin (Sinequan). All of them are hydrochlorides and so all of them have the term after the first word in the chemical labeling; for example, amitriptyline hydrochloride.

Another chemical which is very useful in treating the patient with depression and his or her headache pain is the MAO inhibitor. This is a mood elevator that preserves the catecholamines by decreasing their rate of metabolism.

In severe cases, the two kinds of drugs may be prescribed for the same patient. But that can be done only with considerable caution and strictly as a desperation measure with both the physician and patient understanding the likelihood that there may possibly be severe side effects.

How is the headache triggered by anxiety treated?
We may temporarily use mild pain-relieving and tranquilizing drugs; however, it's most important to take steps to find out what the problem is. One very basic way is to try to get the patient talking about his or her life, family, and work. There may be some factor in these elements or in that individual's social or sexual activities that has touched off the headaches. What the doctor is looking for is a stress situation in the patient's life, usually one that he or she does not feel comfortable talking about at home or wherever the stress occurs. If the patient talks it out with the doctor, the doctor not only learns something that is useful in the patient's treatment, but the patient sometimes experiences a relief from pain in the process.

Aren't there any nonchemical ways of treating headaches triggered by anxiety?
For those who want to substitute a more innovative treatment of the patient than chemicals, there's biofeedback. We treat both the patient and the headache. Again, I always recommend psychotherapy for our patients.

Can biofeedback be used with all patients with headaches triggered by depression?
Biofeedback can help some mildly depressed headache patients. However, many will need a combination of the antidepressant drugs and biofeedback.

In any event, we tend to be selective in the kind of person who is exposed to biofeedback. And again, it's more likely to be a young person who yields to treatment. (Anxiety headaches are likely to appear in the old as well as the young.)

Is there any other kind of headache that falls into this category? I've heard people talk about something called a posttraumatic headache.
You're right. A posttraumatic headache is one that follows an injury to the head. A person who cracks his head against the dashboard of a car when the brakes are applied too swiftly and gets a bump so bad that he or she must be hospitalized may develop a posttraumatic headache. I'd say that one-third to one-half of all such people who injure their heads that badly develop posttraumatic headache. In some cases, the headache may be due to some organic aftereffect of the injury—the development of a blood clot in the lining of the brain that gradually becomes large enough to cause pain, for example. That's why we give patients who describe an injury to the head a very thorough physical examination.

In most cases, however, there is no identifiable organic cause of the headache. The brain may very well be injured, or the supporting tissues about the head and neck, but we are not able to pinpoint a definite physical problem. Moreover, depression often can subtly set in and add to the headache. In such cases, the antidepressant drugs are usually effective in helping the headache as well as easing the patient's depression.

You mentioned three basic categories of headache. We've gone through vascular and tension-type headaches. What is the other classification of headache?
It's the secondary headache. It's the kind of headache that is due solely to organic causes; for example, something that has gone physically wrong in the body and often in the head.

Such as...?

289

There are so many things that might go wrong and cause headache as a symptom that it would take an encyclopedia to list them all. But in general, these headaches could be symptoms of blood clots inside the skull, brain tumors, aneurysms, neuralgia, problems of the neck and spine, or problems with the eyes, ears, or even the teeth. The list could, in fact, go on and on to such a length that it would be intimidating, if not frightening.

What can you, as a doctor, do to diagnose my headache problem, particularly when the possible causes are so many and so diverse?
We do what we can to determine the kind of classification of the headache. We don't assume that it's an organically caused headache; we just accept this as one of the possibilities. But the procedure is the same, no matter what kind of headache it turns out to be.

What is that procedure?
The first and most important task is to take a detailed case history from the patient. This case history should include the following items:

- A family medical history; this helps trace the headache as a family factor, as well as other incidents in the family history that may be important.
- A personal medical and surgical history of the patient.
- The allergic history of the patient; this includes not only allergies or sensitivities which might cause headaches, but more importantly, allergies to any of the drugs we might prescribe to relieve the patient's problem.
- The obstetrical and menstrual history of the female patient.
- A history of the headache: its frequency, location, duration, severity, and timing.
- A review of the circumstances that might be associated with the headache: the sleep habits, emotional pitch, bodily changes (as in

290

menstruation), the patient's relationship to his or her job, and the patient's environment (family and otherwise).

- An examination of previous tests made for the headache and the medicines used, past and present, to treat it.

Does all this help find the headache directly? Or is it aimed mostly at record-gathering that may lead indirectly to a solution?
Both. You can see how all this helps indirectly in awakening possibilities or eliminating others.

But there are times when you will get information of a very significant kind. You may find from the patient's medical history that he or she is a diabetic. We know from past research that certain kinds of headache pain, such as migraine, appear to decrease when the victim develops diabetes, so we can begin to eliminate migraine as the kind of headache or we can begin looking at that patient's blood sugar level as being defective, which would be as important to his diabetes as to his headache.

Or you may get information that seems very insignificant and yet leads directly to a way to end the headaches. I can recall once seeing a young boy who complained of a headache that appeared to act very much like a migraine. But it didn't have any regularity akin to migraine; instead, it appeared only spasmodically and capriciously. But through conversation with the boy and his parents about when the headaches come on, I'd hear references to, "Well, it was the day after we went to the ball game..." or "Remember, it was the night of the school picnic..."

I asked if the boy ate hot dogs, or an unusual number of them, on such occasions. In fact, he'd been at a beach outing with the family only a few days earlier—before the latest onset of headaches—and he'd eaten somewhat more than his share of hot dogs.

That was the most important clue I could gather in the whole extended interview. For this youngster had what we call the "hot dog headache."

291

What is the hot dog headache?

This is a vascular headache suffered by people who are sensitive to a compound called sodium nitrite, a chemical used to preserve meat. It is found most often in hot dogs, but it can be found in a good many other preserved meats. The sensitivity often seems to strike people who might be prone to migraine and touches off attacks that are very similar to migraine, except that they don't have the pattern of migraine; they have the pattern of hot dog consumption.

What tests other than a good case history are important in diagnosing the problem of a headache victim?

That's pretty much going to be determined by the insight gained from the patient's history. For example, I didn't feel there was a need for further tests in the case of the boy with the hot dog headache. I just urged the youngster not to eat any more hot dogs. I told him to call me if he got more headaches or come back and see me in two months if he didn't. In that way, I could double-check his condition.

But in most cases, the doctor already has results of the simplest tests: weight, pulse, and blood pressure. The latter can be an important clue, for many persons with high blood pressure also get headaches related to their ailment.

From there we go on to a thorough neurological examination. This is a series of simple tests that can be performed by the doctor in his or her office. For the patient, they may range from standing on one leg and then the other, to touching the tip of his or her nose with the index finger. They may include having the doctor do everything from tapping the knee with a percussion hammer to scraping the soles of the patient's bare feet. Though they are simple, they are very revealing: if the big toe bends upward in the bare foot test instead of curling downward, you raise a suspicion of a disturbance in the brain or the spinal cord.

Beyond this, I'm inclined to order an MRI in most patients, unless the kind and cause of the headache has been identified before getting to this point. There is just a chance that you may turn up signs of a brain tumor—albeit a small chance because they're so rare in headache patients.

We also do a complete blood analysis in our office if the situation demands it.

What is a CAT scan?

This is a test where many X-ray pictures of the head are taken, run through a computer, and reconstructed by it (the amount of radiation involved in a CAT scan is quite small). With this devise, we can safely screen patients for brain tumors and other major problems that may give them headaches. The scans are performed on an outpatient basis and usually only require a few minutes to complete the examination.

I've often heard the word angiogram; what exactly is this test?

Occasionally, a patient is suspected of having an abnormality in a blood vessel, such as an aneurysm or arteriovenous malformation. A CAT scan may not reveal this problem. In these unusual situations, an angiogram will be performed. In this test, dye is injected into the patient's artery by a thin tube called a catheter, and many X-rays are taken as the dye passes through the arteries around the brain. This test has some risks and is not performed very frequently these days. Since 1988 there have been many advances in diagnosis, the major ones being the MRI (magnetic resonance imaging) and MRA (magnetic resonance angiogram).

What is an MRI?

The diagnosis of headache still rests on taking a careful history, performing a thorough examination, and, if necessary, imaging. These tests are performed not so much to make a diagnosis, but rather to make sure that a more serious or organic problem is not responsible for the headache and neurologic symptoms that a headache sufferer experiences. MRI is also known as nuclear magnetic resonance (NMR). These terms refer to the ability to take a picture of the brain by looking at how the atoms in the brain respond to the effects of radio waves within a large magnet. Scientists discovered years ago that every chemical responds a little bit differently to the effects of radio waves when placed in a strong magnetic field; literally, a fingerprint exists for each chemical in nature. This same type of technique applied on a larger scale allows us to take a picture of the brain. Each section of the brain and organic problems within the brain, such as tumors, cysts, blood clots, scar tissue from a stroke, or even the plaques seen in multiple sclerosis, produce their own unique picture on the MRI scan. MRI has helped us to investigate and determine the source of several patients' problems.

A few years back, for example, we saw a young woman who had been to many doctors before coming to us for her headaches. What was most distressing to this woman was not the pain, since it was relatively mild, but rather the fact that she experienced severe nausea and vomiting every several weeks. The nausea and vomiting lasted for days at a time and, as a result, the woman needed to be hospitalized and given intravenous fluids. All our exams, tests, and treatments proved fruitless in explaining the cause of her problem. Finally, we used the MRI, which unfortunately revealed a small tumor located in a portion of the brain called the brain stem. This portion of the brain is the control center for all the nerves of the head—it controls vital functions such as blood pressure, heart rate, and our breathing pattern, and it carries all the messages from the body to the brain and back to the body. In addition, there is a small group of cells that exists in the brain stem, and when these cells are stimulated in a certain fashion, they cause a person to become nauseated and to vomit. The MRI enabled us to find the cause of this patient's problem.

In another patient who was rather elderly, we thought a stroke she had suffered was causing some deterioration of nervous system functioning. Her previous tests had included a CAT scan, brain scan, and even angiograms of the small blood vessels of the brain. All were normal, but her MRI scan revealed a small area of scar tissue that would have occurred because of a stroke right in the area of the brain that controlled the specific functions that had failed in her case. Besides using this test to look for these types of problems, an MRI may also be helpful if a person cannot have a CAT scan because they are severely allergic to the X-ray dye we need to use, or they are susceptible to radiation sickness in which the exposure to X-rays makes them very ill. The magnetic resonance image does not use any type of radiation to make its picture. Instead, it uses magnets and radio waves which are like the type of radio waves that bring us the sound on our radios. Moreover, the test causes no pain, and uses no injections. The most difficult part of the test is the need to lie very still in the rather small opening between the magnets. Recently a more diagnostic test called an MRA has been perfected for the diagnosis of aneurisms in the brain circulation. This involves the injection of a dye with the usual MRI procedure. It has become a life-saving procedure in many cases.

Are spinal taps still used?
Occasionally, if the doctor suspects an aneurysm or meningitis, a spinal tap is performed. Spinal taps do not have the serious side effects that are often feared with this procedure. With the availability of CT and MRI, though, far fewer spinal taps are performed.

How about regular X-rays of the head?
These "plain skull films" are very rarely used today, because of the use of CT and MRI.

What is an EEG?
This is an electroencephalogram, or a brain wave test. Here, the patient lies down and has a machine record his or her brain waves over a one-hour period. It

is harmless, does not hurt, and can occasionally help in the diagnosis of certain headaches and seizures.

In all the talk about headaches, the causes seem to be adult-oriented— dissatisfactions, depressions, anxieties, organic failure. Don't children ever get headaches?

Some of their headaches are caused by classic childhood problems—fever, mumps, measles, infection of the inner ear, eyestrain. Some of the causes have higher implications: children who get headaches when they fall prey to motion sickness, with its nausea, often show a migraine history in the family. Thus, their headaches are, in reality, migraine headaches.

Some childhood headaches have the same source as adult headaches: anxiety. Children may, if they're high achievers, become very anxious about their schoolwork and develop headaches as a result. It's usually the kids who don't care about their studies who don't get headaches over their schoolwork.

Some of the causes may duplicate adult experiences. Adult men and women have been known to suffer chronic, recurring headaches when thrown into a new job situation or when forced to move from a beloved home to live among strangers in a new city. Their children may suffer in the same way: the pressures of moving are not less severe for them, because they're young, than they are for their parents.

Sometimes the cause can be found in imitation of adult experience. A child may see that his or her mother gets out of certain responsibilities around the house—say, washing the dishes—by complaining of a headache. And so, the child learns to use the complaint of a headache to get out of a homework assignment. But children, being infinitely susceptible to suggestion, may find that the headache becomes real.

How do you treat children with headache?

296

On occasion, children can be treated with the same drugs that we use in treating adults, but in milder dosages and perhaps in different combination.

In general, though, I'm likely to select medicines that have less impact on the child. For migraine, my first choice is likely to be cyproheptadine (Periactin), as a preventive medicine. Propranolol is safe and often effective in children.

We prescribe triptans for children, and rizatriptan is FDA-approved to use in children as young as six years old.

In general, we give children the same thoughtful care for their headaches—including an effort to find organic reasons for them—that we give to adults. For if we can reduce the pain and cut off the cause in childhood, we may give the patient the gift of many more years of happy and fulfilling life.

Will you give a narcotic-based drug to a child?

No, never. For one thing, the impact is likely to be too great for a child. For another thing, these drugs are habituating for children as well as adults, and I think that doctors and everyone in the field of medicine must be extraordinarily careful not to get anybody hooked on drugs.

To be sure, there may be times when a physician is justified in prescribing or administering a narcotic for a patient already in the throes of a severe headache. The idea is to kill the pain, and certain narcotics are very effective pain-killers. But this treatment cannot often be repeated for fear that the patient may become dependent on the narcotic.

Similarly, there are other drugs, not clearly labeled as narcotics, which should be used with caution. Certainly, they should not be used daily—in preventive therapy—even by patients with very severe and recurring headache problems. For they often contain barbiturates or other chemicals which the patient, in all innocence, may not know will hook him or her.

Is drug habituation often seen in headache victims?

Often is perhaps too strong a word. But ideally, we shouldn't see it at all. The fact is that headache victims are very tempted to overuse or abuse their medication because they suffer so much pain so regularly. It starts with aspirin; they feel that if they just take enough of it, they'll kill the pain. They're wrong, but they don't know it. They don't even know that aspirin, as we've already seen, can have some ill-effects when taken in excess.

But if they go to a doctor who does not specialize in headaches, they may get a prescription for a drug which they take at first as prescribed. But then they take more and more of the drug in an effort to escape the headache pain, and soon they're abusing it.

At worst, the drug abuse becomes so intense that by the time the patient gets to a headache specialist, particularly if he or she has been taking drugs by injection. And the doctor has the problem of curing not only that individual's headache pain but his or her drug habituation.

How can a patient know if he or she is bordering on an excess of drug intake?

Medication overuse headache, formerly known as rebound headache, can result from the overuse of medications that are meant to be taken on an as-needed basis. The International Headache Society diagnostic criteria for medication overuse define the overuse of medications as more than 10 doses per month for more than three months of the following medications: opioids, combination analgesics (such as Fioricet), triptans, and ergotamine. For NSAIDs such as naproxen and ibuprofen, medication overuse is defined as more than 15 days of use per month for more than three months.

Can you get the patient to admit to taking this much medicine? Isn't this a confession of drug abuse on the patient's part?

You must be subtle in uncovering this information. I mean you just don't go us to a patient and say, "How long have you been abusing this drug?"

But you might say something like, "How long will 100 Excedrin last you?" or "Do you buy Advil in large lots?" A few more questions like that and you'll have a pretty good idea of how much of the medicine the patient is taking.

Do you have any safeguards against your own patients taking too much of a drug?

Yes. Some of our prescriptions for drugs that I believe to be habit-forming are not refillable None of them can be refilled after six months, no matter what the compound.

For those who don't want to be exposed to drugs, even to overcome their headaches, is acupuncture an adequate alternative?

There is evidence that acupuncture can be beneficial in migraine, and it is true that the Chinese have used it for many years for whole series of problems relating to pain. Among these are migraine pain, arthritis, high blood pressure, and glaucoma. (Headache can be a symptom of the latter three ailments.) There is no doubt that in certain medical situations acupuncture seems to work, even though it must be recognized that Eastern Medicine physicians traditionally have not practiced under the guidelines of rigidly controlled scientific studies in the same tradition as we have in the United States and the Western world.

Before starting therapy, headache patients should be assured that their problem has been diagnosed adequately. Also, patients should have also given the conventional methods of treatment a reasonable trial. For example, patients should not consider acupuncture as the ultimate therapy for headaches.

My own experience suggests that acupuncture may help in relieving the pain of a specific headache. I have the feeling that the doctor must be highly selective in prescribing acupuncture to patients. It also should be noted that transcutaneous stimulators have been used and the Cefaly device is now FDA approved for the prevention of migraine. It is worn on the forehead for 20 minutes daily.

One of the most common forms of the headache pain is the hangover. What can the victim of this kind of headache do for the pain?
The simplest, most dramatic remedy for this kind of headache is the obvious one: don't drink. For if hangover headache is a chronic, recurring pain, then the victim has a chronic problem with alcohol. By solving that problem, he or she can solve the hangover problem.

Do you always have to drink a great deal to get a hangover?
There is considerable evidence that even very little alcoholic intake can affect some people quite deeply and leave them with, among other things, a hangover.

What can be done before you start drinking to prevent a hangover?
One idea is to consume the things ahead of time which will allow the ethyl alcohol, a substance found in almost all liquor, to be burned up more rapidly.

A very easy and handy way to do this is to eat some ripe fruit or certain vegetables beforehand or to drink certain vegetable extracts, such as tomato juice, or simply to eat some honey. For all these foods contain a common sugar, fructose. We know, from highly scientific investigations, that the addition of fructose to the diet contributes very materially to the metabolism of ethyl alcohol by the body. And the faster you can metabolize the ethyl alcohol, the less your chance of suffering a devastating hangover the next day.

Is there anything else besides food that can lessen the hangover?
Very definitely. Don't drink a great deal when you're very fatigued or very tense of depressed. That is because the state of the body and the nervous system seems to contribute to the hangover. Indeed, it's wise to take a nap before going out partying at night, just to give the body and the nervous system a rest.

So be aware of your physical, nervous, or mental state before drinking. If you're frustrated by your job or hate your boss and he or she turns up at the party when you've had too much to drink, worrying about what you said at the party can give you a terrible tension headache the next day.

What can you do while you're drinking to prevent hangover?
The obvious thing is to be very aware of what you eat and drink while partying. Usually, there is a dazzling array of hors d'oeuvres at a good cocktail party— canapés, nuts, different kinds of chips and dips, and a great variety of other exotica. Much of this is going to cause your stomach, liver, and gallbladder, all of which are being hit hard by the wash of ethyl alcohol passing through your system, to give up and act wretched the next day.

If you're somewhat selective about what you eat, you can reduce the impact of this problem. Snacking on cheese in sensible amounts should introduce some of the protein that will reduce the irritant effect of the ethyl alcohol on the lining of the stomach. Of course, aged cheese is not recommended for migraines. A thoughtful host will provide honey (fructose) among the hors d'oeuvres. By snacking on the honey, you will find that the alcohol has far less of a hangover effect.

Are some liquors more likely to cause hangovers than others?
That is still a matter of investigation within medicine. But is widely believed that those liquors which are low in congeners offer the best chance of reducing or eliminating the impact of a hangover.

What are congeners?
In the case of alcohol, they are small molecules, other than ethyl alcohol, produced during the fermentation, distillation, and aging of the liquor or wine.

Many of them have their origin in the grain from which the liquor is made. Many more are contained in the wood of the barrels in which the liquor is

301

aged. You tend to find more congeners in the best bourbons and Scotch, for example, because they've been aged in wood for so much longer than cheaper whiskeys.

When the liquor is ready to be sold and consumed, the congeners have given it that particular taste, color, aroma, and even flavor. They have, in fact, given it much of the distinction that classifies it as a whiskey, gin, wine, or other liquor.

For the more scientifically minded, the congeners are the esters, tannin, fusel oils, furfural, aldehydes, and acids—especially acetic acid—found in different liquors. These congeners may themselves be toxic, particularly when taken in very large and concentrated quantities. But you are not likely to get them in such quantities in liquor.

Which liquors have the greatest number of congeners?
As it happens, the number of congeners varies from liquor to liquor. As we've seen, the more expensive and thus most aged bourbon and Scotch will likely have a greater number of congeners than less costly whiskeys, simply because they've been aged in wood for so much longer.

Which is low in congeners?
Vodka is notably low in congeners. That's because it's almost pure grain alcohol and distilled water. It is almost odorless and tasteless, as is ethyl alcohol. One can obviously get quite drunk while drinking vodka, but is said by some investigators that the side effects, particularly hangover, are far less serious than in consuming other liquors.

But I must make a point. If you're thinking of switching from gin martinis to vodka martinis, just remember one thing—the vermouth in the martinis contains congeners. So, a vodka martini is not altogether a safe haven for avoiding hangover.

One the other hand, a Bloody Mary offers a double-barreled advantage. For one thing, the only liquor it has is vodka. For another thing, it offers a goodly does of tomato juice—in the "natural" Bloody Mary—and the tomato juice contains fructose, which itself helps to reduce the hangover effect by allowing the body to metabolize the ethyl alcohol better. (One caution: watch out for the Tabasco sauce. You don't have to load up on it in every drink.)

Are there other ways to ward off hangovers?

When you go home after a night of drinking, eat some honey. Perhaps you may want to spread it on a piece of toast or on some crackers. While you're sleeping, the fructose in the honey will be helping your body to metabolize the alcohol you've consumed and thus reduce some of the hangover experience of the next morning.

What do you do when you wake up with a hangover?

First, you must understand that the hangover is made up of more than a headache. It is usually accompanied by nausea, vomiting, and dehydration.

Complete rest, isolation, and a dark room are the best possible therapy—not to mention an environment where all those ants aren't stomping around and where the dust isn't crashing noisily to the floor.

You've got to deal first with the headache pain. The pain comes from blood vessels in the head that have been enlarged, or dilated, from the impact of alcohol. In other words, this is a vascular headache, one that's akin to the phenomenon of the migraine headache. The pain is a throbbing one, and the throbbing is at the same rate as the pulse. It just happens that the pulse is going at a faster rate than normal because alcohol accelerates the heartbeat and the pulse rate.

The logical thing to do is to reduce the dilation of the blood vessels. The home remedy for that is to drink lots of coffee, because coffee contains caffeine and caffeine causes the blood vessels to constrict.

Are there other problems besides the headache pain in a hangover?

You must tackle the problem of dehydration, for alcohol is a diuretic. It causes you to urinate more often than normal. There's a hormone in the brain that tends to decrease urine flow, and thus conserve water. Alcohol inhibits the work of that brain hormone. Thus, urine flow is not decreased. It is, in fact, considerably increased.

By the time you wake up the next morning with a hangover, your tongue is dry and furry, and the mucous membranes of the mouth are dry and sticky. You know you're dehydrated. What you don't know is that in addition to water, your body has lost certain salts and chemicals.

What can be done for dehydration?

The solution for dehydration is not to suddenly drink a lot of water. The reason is that a large water load in the stomach will tend to increase nausea and vomiting.

The secret is to drink fluids that contain the minerals and salts that help speed absorption into the bloodstream and that offset the dehydration. One such fluid is orange juice. The trouble with drinking it in the early stages of hangover is that it may increase nausea. The citric acids in orange juice may further upset an already unsettled stomach.

A more logical choice is to drink salty broth when you get up. Several cups of beef broth on arising will do much to relieve the overall problem of dehydration. It will not upset the stomach. It will replace certain salts and minerals that the body needs after dehydration. And it will provide water in a way that the body can accept.

After several hours have passed, drink some more beef broth. You will have undoubtedly gone to the bathroom in the hours after arising, and the second consumption of beef broth will again help to replace the necessary salts and chemicals and fluids.

You will find that this is also useful in controlling the nausea. If you can attack the headache and the dehydration, you will likely find that problems of nausea and vomiting are reduced.

What about other home solutions?

One is to apply an ice pack to the head. This has, in fact, some use in helping to constrict the blood vessels of the head. Ice and deep cold usually accomplish the goal.

Another home solution is to apply a tight band around the head. But this does nothing except warn the family that the wearer is in deep distress and that everybody should walk softly.

Why not take another drink?

Some feel that this is still another remedy—"the hair of the dog"—to drink more of whatever made you feel bad in the first place. Basically, this is silly. You can make an argument that the drink will deliver water and certain chemicals back in the system. But it also causes more urination, further irritation of the stomach lining, increased heartbeat and pulse, dilation of the blood vessels of the head, and a general repetition of the problems that are plaguing you because of drinking too much.

Consider the question in a different light: If you'd hurt your thumb very badly slamming it with a hammer, would you get up in the morning and slam it with the hammer once again—all in the expectation that it's going to hasten the healing of the thumb?

Of course not.

And so why would having a "hair of the dog" help to reduce the problem which the liquor prompted in the first place?

How do you really take care of a hangover headache?

In short, taking care of a hangover headache demands nothing more than the application of your intelligence.

You can help to prevent it by what you consume before going out. You can help to prevent or reduce it by what you consume when you're out partying. And you can help to treat it by what you consume when you awaken in the morning—with a memory of what might have been done to avoid the miseries of the day.

You urge that individuals with chronic and recurring headache pain go to a headache specialist to seek help. Where can I find such a specialist?
One source you can contact is the National Headache Foundation, headquartered at 820 N. Orleans St., #411, Chicago, Illinois 60610. The Foundation is a nonprofit organization dedicated to the investigation of headache, head pain, and the nature of the pain itself. It publishes a quarterly newsletter, provides educational programs on headache, and offers advice for headache problems. You can write to the Foundation for a list of its medical members to see if there is one practicing near your locale, or call the NHF at 312.274.2650. You can also visit the NHF website at www.headaches.org.

EPILOGUE

- Dr. Seymour Diamond's first article on headache was written in 1964 when he operated a family practice. It was on headache and depression.

- He was elected to office in the American Association for the Study of Headache (now the American Headache Society) in 1964. He served as Executive Secretary and was a President of the organization.

- Founded National Migraine Foundation in 1970.

- Dr. Seymour Diamond limited his practice to the treatment of headache in 1972.

- The Diamond Headache Clinic, established in 1974, was the first private headache clinic in the U.S.

- The first edition of this book was published in 1974.

- The Diamond In-patient Headache Unit was founded in 1980 and was the first acute hospital headache treatment unit.

- The unit was moved from Methodist Hospital to Weiss Memorial Hospital in 1983, to Columbus Hospital in 1993, and to St. Joseph Hospital in 2000 where it remains today. It is a 49-bed headache in-patient unit.

- The second edition of this book was published in 1988, but before that the first course of the Diamond Headache Clinic Research and Education Foundation was held in Cincinnati in 1987.

- Dr. Merle Diamond joined the practice in 1989 and became a partner in 1991.

- Dr. Merle Diamond became Managing Partner in 2008 and Dr. Seymour Diamond left the practice but retained the title of Director Emeritus and Founder in 2010.

- Dr. Seymour Diamond remains active as Executive Chairman of the National Headache Foundation at the age of 92.

Appendix I
Diamond Headache Clinic Headache History

1. How many types of headache do you experience?

2. When did you first experience a headache? Can you relate it to any event (head injury, infection, surgery, stress, or for women, menses or pregnancy)?

3. How often do you experience a headache?

4. How long does your headache last? If you take a drug for your headache, how long will the headache last?

5. In what part of your head do you feel the pain? Does the pain move around your head? Is the headache always on one side?

6. During a headache, do you feel pain in your neck or shoulders?

7. How would you rate the severity of your headaches on a scale of 1 (least severe) to 10 (most severe)?

8. How would you describe the pain (throbbing, pulsating, tight head-band, deep boring sensation, ache, vise-like)?

9. Do you have any warning that a headache will soon start? Do you see flashing lights or different colors? Do you have problems with your vision (loss of visual field, images look larger or smaller, blurred vision)? Prior to the headache, do you feel hungry, fatigued, loss of appetite, burst of energy, quick tempered?

10. During a headache do you have any associated symptoms (nausea, vomiting, dizziness, sensitivity to light or sound, facial flushing, nasal congestion, runny nose, tearing in either eye, eyelid droopy or swollen, ringing in the ears, blurred vision)?

11. Can you identify any factor that precipitates your headache? Are you affected by certain foods, alcoholic beverages, skipping meals, skipping caffeine beverages, lack of sleep, changes in weather, certain drugs (nitrates, indomethacin), exercise, stress, or for women, menses?

12. How would you describe your sleep pattern? Do you experience difficulty falling asleep or staying asleep? Does the headache awaken you from a sound sleep? Do you awake and find the headache has already started?

13. How would you describe your marital and family relationships? Are you under stress at home or at work? For children and adolescents, are you under stress at school? Have you missed work of school days because of the headaches?

14. What are you medical and surgical histories? Have you ever been hospitalized for headaches?

15. For women: What is your menstrual history? At what age did your periods start? Did you have headaches during your pregnancy? Are you on birth control pills or hormone supplements?

16. What medications do you use for your headaches? Are you on preventive medications for headaches? What medications have you previously tried for headaches?

17. Are you on medications for any other medical condition?

18. Are you allergic to any medications? Do you have seasonal allergies? Do you have any food allergies?

19. How many cups of coffee, tea, or caffeine-containing soda do you drink per day?

20. Do you smoke?

21. Do you drink alcoholic beverages on a daily basis? How often do you drink?

22. Do you use any recreational drugs?

23. Have you ever tried alternative therapies for your headaches (biofeedback, acupuncture, massage)?

24. Are you using any herbal remedies for your headaches?

25. Have you had any recent tests because of your headaches? Have you ever received neuroimaging (CT scan or MRI) because of your headaches?

Adapted from Headache *and Migraine Biology and Management,* published by Elsevier Science and Technology Books, Chapter 3, with permission from Edmund Messina, Michigan Headache Clinic, East Lansing, Michigan.

Appendix II
Efficacy of Acute Treatment Based on Headache Phase

Medication	Vulnerability phase	Premonitory phase	Mild headache phase	Moderate to severe headache phase	Rescue phase	Postdrome phase
Sumatriptan SC			++++	====	+++	
Parenteral triptans; nasal and transdermal			++++	+++	++	
Oral triptans	Frovatriptan	Frovatriptan	++++	++	+	Likely beneficial
	Sumatriptan	Naratriptan				
	Zolmitriptan					
Sumatriptan/naproxen	Likely beneficial	Likely beneficial*	++++	+++	++	Likely beneficial
Diclofenac powder	Likely beneficial	Likely beneficial*	++++	+++	++	Likely beneficial
Antiemetics alone or in combination				+++	+++	
Dihydroergotamine IV	+++	+++	+++	+++	+++	
Opioids				++	+++	
Phenothiazines			+++	+++	+++	
Metopropramide			++	++	++	
Chlorpromazine				+++	+++	

*Adapted from Bedell AW, et al. Patient-centered Strategies for effective management of migraine. Primary Care Network, 2000. Level of efficacy: + Somewhat, ++ Mild, +++ Moderate, ++++ High

Adapted from *Headache and Migraine Biology and Management*, published by Elsevier Science and Technology Books, Chapter 8, with permission from Roger K. Kady and Kathleen Farmer, Headache Care Center, Springfield, Missouri.

Appendix III
Migraine Preventive Therapy: What's in the Pipeline?

The American Migraine Prevalence and Prevention (AMPP) study showed that only 13 percent of migraine patients were receiving preventive therapy, while 38 percent of migraine patients could have potentially benefited from it. The US Headache Consortium guidelines suggested that migraine patients with six or more headache days per month should be offered preventive therapy, and they also suggested that those with three to four headache days per month should be offered this therapy if there is significant functional disability.

So why is migraine preventive therapy so severely underutilized? To understand this we must look at what options are currently available and realize what their shortcomings may be.

The first medication specifically designed as a migraine preventive medication was methysergide. This was an extremely effective medication for migraine prevention, but it unfortunately had significant complications in the form for pulmonary and retroperitoneal fibrosis that could severely complicate lung and kidney function. In addition, there was some significant vascular risk associated with this compound. These issues have resulted in methysergide being removed from the U.S. market (although it still is available in some foreign countries).

Until now, subsequent preventive medications that have been used were all originally introduced for other medical indications and found to be effective for migraine prevention after their introduction to the U.S. market. These include a variety of medications used for epilepsy (topiramate, valproate and gabapentin), hypertension (propranolol, metoprolol, timolol, verapamil, lisinopril, and candesartan) and depression (amitriptyline, nortriptyline, and venlafaxine). OnabotulinumtoxinA (Botox) is also commonly used for patients meeting criteria for chronic migraine. These are just some of the more commonly tried preventive agents. All are limited in varying degrees by tolerability issues, even when good efficacy may be present.

So what does the future hold? Are there therapies being developed that are migraine-specific? Are there therapies "already out there" that may be of value for migraine prevention?

Here are some of the areas of current research interest:

Calcitonin gene related peptide (CGRP)

Monoclonal antibodies: targeting the receptor cell or the CGRP ligand itself

Small molecules targeting the receptor

Combination drugs or new delivery systems

Dextromethorphan/quinidine

Oxytocin nasal spray

New neurostimulators

Vagus nerve

Sphenopalatine ganglion

Supraorbital

Temporo-auricular

Occipital

Transcutaneous magnetic (TMS)

There are several reasons why CGRP modulation is currently such a hot area of migraine research. CGRP is an excitatory and inflammatory neurotransmitter released from trigeminovascular sensory nerve cells. It is a potent dilator of blood vessels. It causes extravasation of inflammatory plasma proteins and increases pain transmission in both the peripheral and central nervous systems. Levels of CGRP are elevated in the blood, spinal fluid, and saliva of migraine patients. When injected intravenously, CGRP induces migraine-like headaches in susceptible individuals.

CGRP monoclonal antibodies are currently the most exciting potential preventive agents being studied. There are four of these currently in Phase III clinical trials. All seem to be faring well in terms of efficacy and tolerability based on the Phase II data and early Phase III studies. CGRP is an extremely important player in the migraine process. It plays a role in vasodilation, inflammation, and pain transmission. Triptans work acutely by stimulating the 5-HT1 B, D and F receptors. By stimulating the D receptor, they inhibit the release of CGRP. It is felt that this reduces not only vasodilation, but also inflammation and pain transmission. The effect of this is short-lived, so these are used almost exclusively for acute migraine abortive therapy. It is also felt that onabotulinumtoxinA may be working at least in part in the preventive therapy of chronic migraine by the prolonged inhibition of CGRP release for about 12 weeks.

Biologic agents such as CGRP monoclonal antibodies are manufactured in the laboratory starting with antibodies made in nonhuman species (such as mice or rats). Individual components of these nonhuman immunoglobulins are then gradually substituted for, making them humanized (90-percent human) or even fully humanized (100-percent human). This reduces the risks of immunological reactions against them that could either inactivate them or cause allergic reactions. These antibodies also have a long half-life, allowing them be administered monthly or possibly even at three-month intervals. At this time, three of these potential therapeutic agents are being administered as a subcutaneous (SC) injection that will hopefully be easily self-administered by patients. The fourth is an intravenous (IV) preparation that will be administered in an infusion suite by a nurse.

Another group of potential therapeutic agents for migraine prevention are referred to as gepants. These are small molecules (in comparison to antibodies) that block the CGRP receptor cells. The first of these to go through Phase III testing was telcagepant. This showed efficacy both as an abortive agent for acute attacks and as a preventive agent. Unfortunately, it had liver

315

toxicity and never became commercially available. Other agents in this class are currently in clinical trials for both acute and preventive therapy. These appear to have no evidence of liver toxicity. Hopefully, this will hold up through clinical trials.

A combination drug is also currently undergoing clinical trials. This contained a mixture of dextromethorphan and quinidine. It is thought that this might have efficacy based on its effect against glutamate, an excitatory neurotransmitter that is important in the migraine process. It also could be working through modulation of sodium, potassium, and calcium channels. At this point, however, it is too early to tell if this will be of major benefit. There already is substantial data suggesting good tolerability, as it is already commercially available as a treatment for pseudobulbar affect.

Another investigational product being evaluated is a nasal spray of oxytocin. Oxytocin receptors are often found in the company of CGRP receptors in the trigeminal system. Early studies suggest that this may someday be an effective preventive therapy.

Other investigational products are also in early testing. Histamine dihydrochloride is a product planned to be used by SC injection. Magnesium L-lactate dehydrate (MLD10) taken daily is also in early testing.

Various devices are also currently being investigated and evaluated. A hand held vagal nerve stimulator and transcranial magnetic stimulation are noninvasive options in the pipeline that are already being used for migraine prevention as well as for acute therapy. Occipital nerve, supraorbital nerve, and temporo-auricular nerve stimulation are also being used but require surgical implantation and are considered at this time to be "investigational." Likewise, a sphenopalatine ganglion (SPG) implantable stimulator is currently being investigated for chronic cluster headache. Could this also in the future be considered for prophylaxis of intractable chronic migraine? In addition, an intranasal kinetic oscillation stimulation device is being evaluated.

316

In summary, we have found in the last few years that investigational drugs and devices are being increasingly evaluated for migraine prevention. At Island Neurological, we are currently involved in the clinical trials of several of these pharmaceutical products and devices. Since none of the current commercially available products are effective and tolerable for all migraine patients who need them, any new additions that become commercially available are always eagerly awaited by our patients. It remains most important, however, to remember that these patients first need to be properly diagnosed as having migraine. They also need to then be evaluated to decide if preventive therapy is needed in addition to properly utilized acute migraine-specific therapy. Overuse of acute medications must also always be guarded against.

Suggested reading:

- Lipton RB, et al. Migraine prevalence, disease burden, and the need for preventive therapy. *Neurology* 2007;68:343-349.
- Silberstein SD, et al. Evidence-based guideline update: Pharmacologic treatment for episodic migraine prevention in adults. *Neurology* 2012; 78:1337-1345.
- Silberstein SD, et al. Therapeutic monoclonal antibodies: What headache specialists need to know. *Headache* 2015; 55: 1171-1182.

From *Headwise* magazine
Reprinted with permission:
Ira M. Turner, MD, The Center for Headache Care and Research, Island Neurological, ProHealthcare Associates,
Plainview, NY

Appendix IV
Acute Medications for Migraine

Generic Treatment	Doses
Aspirin tablets	325 mg to 650 mg
Acetaminophen	325 mg to 1,000 mg
Combination Analgesics	
Aspirin plus acetaminophen plus caffeine tablets	250 mg plus 250 mg plus 65 mg
Isometheptene mucate plus acetaminophen plus dichloralphenazone tablets	65 mg plus 325 mg plus 100 mg
Butalbital plus aspirin plus caffeine tablets	50 mg plus 325 mg plus 40 mg
Butalbital plus acetaminophen plus caffeine tablets	50 mg plus 325 mg plus 40 mg
Ergotomine alkaloids	
Ergotomine tartrate plus caffeine tablet	1 mg plus 100 mg
Ergotomine tartrate plus caffeine suppository	2 mg plus 100 mg
DHE nasal spray	0.5 mg per nostril (repeat in 15 minutes for a 2 mg total dose)
DHE IM or SC	1 mg
Neuroleptics and Antiemetics	
Chloropromazine capsule	10 mg to 25 mg
Metoclopramide IV	10+ mg
Prochlorperazine	25 mg
NSAIDs	
Diclofenac K tablets	50 mg to 100 mg
Diclofenac potassium	50 mg
Flurbiprofen tablets	100 mg to 300 mg
Ibuprofen tablets	200 mg to 1,200 mg
Naproxen sodium tablets	550 mg to 1,100 mg
Naproxen tablets	250 mg to 500 mg
Piroxicam tablets	40 mg
Tolfenamic acid tablets	200 mg to 400 mg
Opiate Analgesics	
Butorphanol nasal spray	1 to 2 mg
Triptans	
Almotriptan tablets	12.5 mg
Naratriptan tablets	1 mg or 2.5 mg
Rizatriptan tablets	5 mg or 10 mg
Rizatriptan orally disintegrating tablets	5 mg or 10 mg
Sumatriptan tablets	25 mg, 50 mg or 100 mg
Sumatriptan nasal spray	5 mg or 20 mg
Sumatriptan SC self-injection	6 mg
Zolmitriptan tablets	2.5 mg or 5 mg
Zolmitriptan orally disintegrating tablets	2.5 mg or 5 mg

Appendix V
Headache Calendar

Patient's Name _____

Date of Birth _____

Physician's Name _____

Date	Time Onset Ending		Headache Severity	Psychic & Physical Factors	Food & Drink Excesses	Medication Taken & Doses	Headache Relief

Headache Keys

Headache Severity Scale

1		5		10
None	Mild		Moderate	Severe

Psychic & Physical Factors

1. Emotional Upset/Family or Friends
2. Emotional Upset/Occupation
3. Business/Reversal
4. Business/Success
5. Vacation Days
6. Weekends
7. Strenuous Exercise
8. Strenuous Labor
9. High Altitude Location
10. Anticipation Anxiety
11. Crisis/Serious
12. Post-Crisis Period
13. New Job/Position
14. New Move
15. Menstrual Days
16. Physical Illness
17. Over-Sleeping
18. Weather
19. Fasting
20. Missing a Meal
21. Other _____

Food and Drink Excesses

1. Ripened Cheeses (Pizza)
2. Herring
3. Chocolate
4. Vinegar, Fermented Foods (Pickled or Marinated, Sour Cream/Yogurt
5. Freshly Baked Yeast Products
6. Nuts (Peanut Butter)
7. Monosodium Glutamate (MSG—Chinese Food)
8. Pods of Broad Beans
9. Onions
10. Canned Figs
11. Citrus Foods
12. Bananas
13. Pork
14. Caffeinated Beverages (Cola)
15. Avocado
16. Fermented Sausage (Cured Cold Cuts)
17. Chicken Livers
18. Wine
19. Alcohol
20. Beer

Headache Relief Scale

1_____5_____10

None   Mild   Moderate   Severe

Patients on Nardil and/or Marplan should follow the original diet given to them.

Appendix VI
Diamond Headache Clinic's Diet Plan

Low-Tyramine Headache Diet*
Tyramine is produced in foods from the natural breakdown of the amino acid tyrosine. Tyramine is not added to foods. Tyramine levels increase in foods when they are aged, fermented, stored for long periods of time, or are not fresh.

Food group	Allowed	Avoid	Use with caution
Meat, Fish, Poultry, Eggs	Freshly purchased and prepared meats, fish, and poultry Eggs Tuna fish, tuna salad (with allowed ingredients)	Bacon*, sausage*, hot dogs*, corned beef*, bologna*, ham*, any luncheon meats with nitrates or nitrites added. Meats with tenderizer added, caviar	Aged, dried, fermented, salted, smoked, or pickled products. Pepperoni, salami, and liverwurst. Nonfresh meat or liver, pickled herring
Dairy	Milk: whole, 2% or skim Cheese: American, cottage, farmer, ricotta, cream cheese, Velveeta, low-fat processed	Yogurt, buttermilk, sour cream: ½ cup per day Parmesan* or Romano* as a garnish (2 tsp.) or minor ingredient	Aged cheese: blue, brick, brie cheddar, Swiss, Roquefort, stilton, mozzarella, provolone, emmentaler, etc.
Breads, Cereals, Pasta	Commercially prepared yeast Product leavened with baking powder: biscuits, pancakes, coffee	Homemade yeast leavened breads and coffee cakes Sourdough breads	Any with a restricted ingredient

Food group	Allowed	Avoid	Use with caution
	cakes, etc. All cooked and dry cereals All pasta: spaghetti, rotini ravioli, (w/allowed ingredients), macaroni, and egg noodles		
Vegetables	Asparagus, string beans, beets, carrots, spinach, pumpkin, tomatoes, squash, zucchini, broccoli, potatoes, onions cooked in food, Chinese pea pods, navy beans, soy beans, any not on restricted list	Raw onion	Snow peas, fava or broad beans, sauerkraut, pickles, and olives Fermented soy products like miso, soy sauce, and teriyaki sauce
Fruits	Apple, applesauce, cherries, apricots, peaches, any not on restricted list	Limit intake to ½ cup per day from each group: Citrus: orange, grapefruit, tangerine, pineapple, lemon and lime Avocados, banana, figs*, raisins*, dried fruit*, papaya, passion fruit, and red plums	
Nuts and Seeds			All nuts:

Food group	Allowed	Avoid	Use with caution
			peanuts, peanut butter, pumpkin seeds, sesame seeds, walnuts, pecans
Soups	Soups made from allowed ingredients, homemade broths	Canned soups with autolyzed or hydrolyzed yeast*, meat extracts*, or monosodium glutamate* (MSG)	
Beverages	Decaffeinated coffee, fruit juices, club soda, caffeine-free carbonated beverages	Limited caffeinated beverages to no more than 2 servings per day: Coffee and tea: 1 cup = 1 serving carbonated beverages and hot cocoa or chocolate milk: 12oz = 1 serving Limit alcoholic beverages to one serving: 4oz Riesling wine, 1.5 oz vodka or Scotch per day = 1 serving per day (May need to omit if on MAOI)	Alcoholic beverages: Chianti, sherry, burgundy, vermouth, ale, beer, and nonalcoholic fermented beverages. All others not specified in caution column

Food group	Allowed	Avoid	Use with caution
Ingredients Listed on Food Labels	Any not listed in the restricted section		MSG* (in large amounts), nitrates and nitrites (found mainly in processed meats), yeast, yeast extracts, brewer's yeast, hydrolyzed or autolyzed yeast, meat extracts, meat tenderizers (papain, bromelin) seasoned salt (containing MSG), soy sauce, teriyaki sauce
Fats, Oils, and Miscellaneous	All cooking oils and fats White vinegar Commercial salad dressing with allowed ingredients All spices not listed in restricted ingredients	Wine, apple, or other fermented vinegars*	

Carbonated beverages 12oz = 30-50mg (Regular and sugar-free)
Caffeine Content of Selected Beverages
Coffee 6oz = 103mg
Decaffeinated coffee 6oz = 2mg
Tea 6oz = 31-36mg (Instant and 3-minute brew)

General Guidelines

- Each day eat three meals with a snack at night or six small meals spread throughout the day.
- Avoid eating high sugar foods on an empty stomach, when excessively hungry, or in place of a meal.
- All food, especially high protein foods, should be prepared and eaten fresh. Be cautious of leftovers held for more than one or two days at refrigerator temperature. Freeze leftovers that you want to store for more than two or three days.
- Cigarette and cigar smoke contain a multitude of chemicals that will trigger or aggravate your headache. If you smoke, make quitting a high priority. Enter a smoking cessation program.
- The foods listed in the "CAUTION" column have smaller amounts of Tyramine or other vasoactive compounds. Foods with an * may contain small amounts of Tyramine. Other foods in the "USE WITH CAUTION" column do not contain Tyramine but are potential headache "triggers". If you are taking an MAO inhibitor (Monoamine Oxidase Inhibitor) you should test the use of restricted foods in limited amounts.
- Each person may have different sensitivities to certain level of Tyramine or other vasoactive compounds in foods. If you are not on an MAO inhibitor, you should test the use of restricted foods in limited amounts.

*Adapted from the Columbus Hospital & Diamond Headache Clinic Low-Tyramine Headache Diet.

Appendix VII
Nardil Diet (When Taking Monoamine Oxidase Medicines)

Nardil and Marplan are monoamine oxidase inhibitors (MAOIs) which are effective preventive agents in the treatment of headaches. These medications do, however, prevent the body from breaking down a naturally occurring food substance: TYRAMINE. Several foods and beverages contain tyramine and many interact with your medication.

Tyramine is a natural breakdown product of the amino acid tyrosine. Generally it will tend to accumulate in protein containing foods as they age. It is never added to foods, so it will not be included in ingredient lists. You, therefore, need to be aware of the type of foods and storage conditions that need to be avoided to prevent excess tyramine from accumulating in your system.

As always, in the prevention and treatment of headaches it is important to eat a well-balanced and varied diet with at least three meals per day. The information that follows will not interfere with your need of ability to nourish yourself properly.

All foods must be fresh or properly frozen. Avoid foods when you are unaware of storage conditions, especially high-protein foods. In addition, if you purchase or prepare foods, especially meats, fish, and poultry that you will not use up within one to three days, freeze the item to avoid tyramine buildup. Normal shelf life for unopened canned goods is acceptable.

This diet MUST be followed from the day you start taking the medication until two weeks after stopping it.

In addition, please be aware that some foods allowed on the MAOI diet MAY prove to be headache triggers for you.

WHAT IS TYRAMINE?
Tyramine is produced in foods from the natural breakdown of the amino acid tyrosine. Tyramine is not added to foods. Tyramine levels increase

in foods when they are aged, fermented, stored for long periods of time, or are not fresh.

General Guidelines
- Each day eat three meals with a snack at night or six small meals spread throughout the day.
- Avoid eating high sugar foods on an empty stomach, when excessively hungry, or in place of a meal.
- All food, especially high protein foods, should be prepared and eaten fresh. Be cautious of leftovers held for more than one or two days at refrigerator temperature. Freeze leftovers that you want to store for more than two or three days.
- Cigarette and cigar smoke contain a multitude of chemicals that will trigger or aggravate your headache. If you smoke, make quitting a high priority. Enter a smoking cessation program.
- The foods listed in the "CAUTION" column have smaller amounts of Tyramine or other vasoactive compounds. Foods with an * may contain small amounts of Tyramine. Other foods in the "USE WITH CAUTION" column do not contain Tyramine but are potential headache "triggers". If you are taking an MAO inhibitor (Monoamine Oxidase Inhibitor) you should test the use of restricted foods in limited amounts.
- Each person may have different sensitivities to certain level of Tyramine or other vasoactive compounds in foods. If you are not on an MAO inhibitor, you should test the use of restricted foods in limited amounts.

*Adapted from the Columbus Hospital & Diamond Headache Clinic Low-Tyramine Headache Diet.

328

	Food to avoid	Food allowed
Cheese	Cheddar cheese	Fresh cheeses: cottage cheese, cream cheese, ricotta cheese, mozzarella, and processed cheese slices. Aged cheeses (except cheddar) up to 4 oz. per meal.
Meats	Fermented sausage: pepperoni, salami, mortadella, summer sausage, etc. Improperly stored pickled herring, improperly stored meat, fish, poultry	All fresh or frozen meat, fish , or poultry. Lunch meats up to 4 oz. per meal. Store in a refrigerator immediately and eat as soon as possible (or freeze).

Limit any combination of aged cheese and lunch meats to a total of 4 oz. per meal.

	Food to avoid	Food allowed
Fruits and Vegetables	Fava beans, banana peel	All other beans, panama pulp, all others except those listed opposite.
Alcoholic Beverages	All tap beers	No more than TWO domestic bottled or canned beers or 4 oz. of red or white wine per day; this also applies to nonalcoholic beer. Please note that red wine may produce headache unrelated to a rise in blood pressure.
Miscellaneous Foods	Marmite and vegemite concentrated yeast extract	Other yeast extracts (e.g., brewer's years). Soy milk, soy flour, soy cheeses, textured soy protein. Soy sauce and other soybean condiments up to 1 oz. Tofu and tempeh up to 10 oz.

Appendix VIII
Progressive Relaxation Exercises

Let all your muscles go loose and heavy. Just settle back quietly and comfortably ... Wrinkle up your forehead now; wrinkle and smooth it out. Picture the entire forehead and scalp becoming smoother as the relaxation increases ... Now frown and crease your brows and study the tension ... Let go of the tension again, smooth out the forehead once more ... Now, close your eyes tighter and tighter. Feel the tension ... Now relax your eyes. Keep your eyes closed, gently, comfortably, and notice the relaxation ... Now clench your jaws. Bite your teeth together; study the tension throughout the jaws ... Relax your jaws now. Let your lips part slightly ... Appreciate the relaxation.

Now press your tongue hard against the roof of your mouth. Look for the tension ... All right, let your tongue return to a comfortable and relaxed position ... Now purse your lips, press your lips together tighter and tighter ... Relax the lips. Note the contrast between tension and relaxation. Feel the relaxation all over your face, all over your forehead and scalp, eyes, jaws, lips, tongue, and your neck muscles ... Press your head back as far as it can go and feel the tension in the neck. Roll it to the right and feel the tension shift ... Now roll it to the left ... Straighten your head and bring it forward and press your chin against your chest. Let your head return to a comfortable position, and study the relaxation. Let the relaxation develop.

Shrug your shoulders right up. Hold the tension. Drop your shoulders and feel the relaxation. Neck and shoulders are relaxed ... Shrug your shoulders again and move them around. Bring your shoulders up and forward and back. Feel the tension in your shoulders and in your upper back. Drop your shoulders once more and relax. Let the relaxation spread deep into the shoulders, right into your back muscles. Relax your neck and throat, and your jaws and other facial areas as the pure relaxation takes over and grows deeper ... deeper ... ever deeper.

Appendix IX
Temperature Controlling Exercises

The patient receiving temperature feedback training first uses a temperature monitor at home for four weeks. The patient practices twice daily, using the phrases listed below. These are known as autogenic phrases and formulated by Dr. Johannes Schultz.

I feel quiet ... I am beginning to feel quite relaxed ... my feet feel heavy and relaxed ... my ankles, my knees, and my hips feel heavy, relaxed, and comfortable ... my solar plexus and the whole central portion of my body feel relaxed and quiet ... my hands, my arms, and my shoulders feel heavy, relaxed, and comfortable ... my neck, my jaw, and my forehead feel relaxed ... my whole body feels quiet, heavy, comfortable, and relaxed.

Appendix X
Headache Glossary

Abdominal migraine: A type of migraine, in which the pain is over the upper part of the abdomen and lasts a few hours. It is most common in female children. Diagnosis is easily made because of the family history of migraine, the infrequency of the attacks, and the frequent simultaneous occurrence of headache. If it remains undiagnosed, however, the patient may be subjected to unnecessary surgery for abdominal complaints. (*See also migraine equivalent.*)

Acoustic neuroma: A nonmalignant, slow-growing tumor involving the eighth cranial nerve. Headache is a late symptom of this disorder. Other symptoms include dizziness, loss of balance, nausea, and ringing in the ears. Once the headache develops, it grows progressively worse. Diagnosis is very simply made by MRI of the internal auditory canal. Most cases can be adequately treated, with the tumor removed by microsurgery (surgery performed with the aid of an operating microscope).

Acupuncture: An ancient Chinese procedure which blocks pain by stimulating nerves. It is based on the theory that a counterirritant (puncturing) prevents the painful impulses from traveling up the spinal cord and thereby blocks them.

Acute posttraumatic headache: Headache that develops within seven days of head trauma but resolves within three months.

Aging: With age, there is usually a decrease in the number of migraine attacks. Many migraine with aura patients will exhibit only the aura or warning as they grow older.

Alcohol headache: A headache brought on by consumption of alcohol, a vasodilator, which causes the blood vessels of the head to swell. Migraine or cluster headache patients often list alcohol as a precipitating factor. A hangover from alcohol, occurring six hours or later after a drinking bout is probably not due to the immediate effect of drinking alcohol but to the breakdown products when alcohol is metabolized. Alcohol can also contain many impurities known as congeners, which can cause the "hangover headache."

Alice in Wonderland syndrome: A vision of distorted figures of shapes that occurs as part of the migraine attack in certain sufferers. Lewis Carroll got many of his ideas for his book on Alice from the aura he experienced with his migraines.

Allergies: Headache patients may note an increase in headaches during or following an allergic episode because of the acute swelling of the nasal lining and accompanying passages. However, studies have tended to disprove the many claims of a relationship between allergies and headache.

Altitude headache: A headache that develops with travel to a higher altitude. The headache is severe and often mimics migraine. Change in altitude may also increase the frequency of migraine and precipitate an attack. The diuretic acetazolamide (Diamox) can be effective in preventing altitude headache.

Alpha blockers: Drugs that block the effects of adrenalin-related substances on the blood vessel walls and prevent the initial clamping down or vasoconstriction of the blood vessels, thus blocking migraine attacks.

Amines: Biological substances that are normally present in the brain and body and affect blood level functions. Some are found in foods, while others are produced by the body itself. Amines are known to affect mood behavior and blood vessel constriction or swelling.

Amitriptyline: A tricyclic antidepressant frequently used in the prevention of migraine. It has some sedative effect and is often effective in chronic pain syndromes.

Amphetamines: A group of drugs having a stimulant action on the central nervous system. They were used at one time in combination with aspirin and other analgesics to treat migraine. Most headache experts have not found it effective in the treatment of migraine.

Analgesics: Drugs that reduce the perception of pain by raising the patient's pain threshold. They are not cures for pain; they simply mask it. Analgesics range from plain aspirin or acetaminophen (Tylenol, Datril, and so forth) to narcotics like morphine and hydrocodone.

Anaphylaxis: A severe allergic reaction in which the person goes into vascular collapse following the injection or ingestion of a substance to which he or she is sensitive. Symptoms include extreme irritability, shortness of breath, convulsions, loss of consciousness, and shock. Death may result. It is primarily caused by a contraction of the smooth muscle fibers. Rapid action by drugs such as adrenalin and steroids can prevent it. Severe allergic reactions like this rarely result from medicines used in treating migraine, but they may occur as a result of the dyes injected into the blood stream to visualize blood vessels in procedures such as arteriograms or computerized axial scans. A person with a previous history of allergies should be observed very carefully when using certain medications and during certain diagnostic procedures.

Aneurysm: A weakness in the blood vessel wall that balloons out and may rupture at some point. Aneurysms rarely cause symptoms before the rupture, unless they are large. They do not mimic the symptoms of migraine or cluster headache. It is vital to discover them before they rupture and have catastrophic consequences such as paralysis or death. (*See also cerebral aneurysm.*)

Angioma (arteriovenous malformation): A hereditary type of blood vessel tumor consisting of intertwining arteries and veins. The occurrence of the malformation does not appear to be more common in migraine sufferers than in the general population. There have, however, been reports of long-term remissions of migraine attacks in patients who have had large angiomas removed.

Antidepressants: Medications that raise the spirits of seriously depressed people. They focus on the emotion center of the brain and increase its use of certain chemicals present in the brain. Antidepressants elevate the level of the amines that are deficient in various mood and behavioral abnormalities. They may also have a beneficial effect in certain headache problems even when depression is not present.

335

Antiemetic: A drug used to prevent nausea and vomiting. It can be given orally, by injection, or rectally. Most of the drugs used as antiemetics are phenothiazines.

Arteritis: A condition in which there is an inflammation of the blood vessels, often accompanied by vague muscle aches and pains. It occurs most often after age 55. If headaches occur in an older person for the first time, a condition such as arteritis must be considered. Early diagnosis is imperative since early treatment with steroids can prevent the secondary effect of the inflammation of the blood vessels—irreversible blindness. (*See also temporal arteritis.*)

Arthritis: Arthritis of the neck area or cervical spine can be a cause of headache. Imaging of the cervical spine will reveal some changes. If there is limited neck movement, plus articular crepitus (or grating of the neck), and pain in the neck and back of the head if present, arthritis should be suspected.

Asian restaurant syndrome: A condition named for the presence in Asian foods of monosodium glutamate (MSG), which may produce a generalized instability of the blood vessels and thus cause headache, head sweating, or excessive abdominal cramps. Large amounts of monosodium glutamate should be avoided by patients who suffer frequent headaches. (*See also MSG headache.*)

Atherosclerosis: A hardening of the arteries, in particular, a hardening of the arteries of the blood vessels supplying the brain. It can cause some symptoms of headache in the elderly.

Aura: Symptoms that may occur 30 minutes to one hour before the pain of migraine. Auras can be positive, as in vision of bright lights or stars, or lines resembling forts (known as fortification spectra), or they can be negative, as in seeing blind spots or only part of the visual field. Auras may also distort figures or shapes. (*See Alice in Wonderland syndrome.*) Some people get tingling, pins-and-needles sensations in one arm or leg (paresthesias). Some describe a strange odor. All of these are the aura of migraine.

Barbiturates: A group of drugs that act as sedatives and are markedly habituating. Many popular headache medications contain a barbiturate. The primary objection to the use of these drugs is the possibility of addiction if the patient is taking these pains relievers daily, as well as the risk of medication overuse headache.

Basilar type migraine: A type of migraine that can occur in younger people, with the headache most often limited to the back of the head. The symptoms are caused by a diminished blood supply to the parts of the brain supplied by the basilar artery. Besides nausea, patients may have double-vision, unsteady gait, slurred speech, and may seem confused. During the acute headache, many lose consciousness. Often these patients are mistakenly thought to be drunk or mentally ill. A previous history of migraine is helpful in making the diagnosis.

BC-105 (Pizotifen, Sandomigraine): A drug related to the tricyclic antidepressants. It is widely used outside the United States for the treatment of migraine. Careful testing in the United States has not revealed significant results.

Benzodiazepines: Medications that lessen anxiety, emotions, and tension. Many are habituating and, if used in elderly people, can cause some serious side effects.

Beta blockers: A group of drugs that block the action of adrenalin and its byproducts. Since adrenalin is produced by stress and affects the reactivity of the blood vessels, the use of these blocking drugs can be of some help in stress-related migraine. Propranolol (Inderal) is the beta blocker most commonly used in the prevention of migraine.

Biofeedback: A method of treatment in which one is taught to control the body by feeding back the results of performance. With humans, the feedback is artificially mediated by man-made detection, amplification, and display instrumentation rather than being present as an inborn feedback loop within the biological system.

337

Biogenic amines: A group of substances that may control the brain's emotional status.

Blood patch: Procedure in which an injection of the patient's own blood into the site of a spinal puncture used in the treatment of post-spinal puncture headache. After a spinal puncture, whether it is performed for diagnostic purposes or as a method of anesthesia, headache is a frequent complication, and has been a difficult condition to prevent and treat.

BOTOX: *See onabotulinumtoxinaA.*

Brain abscess: Although rare, infection at any site in the body can be carried by the circulatory system to the brain and then develop in the brain or in the tissues surrounding the brain. When this occurs, it may remain dormant for many weeks or even years. Eventually, as the infection grows, the person will develop neurological symptoms. A brain abscess is often masked and may remain undiagnosed. It may result from infections of the sinuses and teeth, tubercular infections of the lungs, or minor skin infections. Differential diagnosis is made through the progression of symptoms, with headache and other neurological manifestations usually becoming progressively worse.

Calcitonin gene-related peptide (CGRP): A neuropeptide that plays a role in the initiation and transmission of, and heightened sensitivity to, migraine pain. New medications which target the action of CGRP are being developed with very encouraging results in clinical trials.

Calcium channel blockers: Blood pressure medications that exert their effect on smooth muscle found in blood vessels as well as the heart. Some calcium channel blockers, including verapamil, have utility in cluster headache and migraine prevention.

Caffeine: A chemical substance naturally occurring in coffee, tea, and cola drinks. It is often combined with analgesics as well as ergotamine tartrate. Indeed, when combined with ergotamine, small amounts of caffeine are often helpful as a synergist in aborting migraine attacks. Excessive amounts of caffeine, however, can increase the number of headaches. Withdrawal from caffeine, as on weekends, can cause the "weekend headache."

Carotid angiogram: A procedure in which dye is injected into the carotid artery, a blood vessel located in the neck, to visualize the circulation in the head as well as in the brain itself. Angiograms were used frequently before the invention of the CT scan. Carotid angiography is also helpful in determining a decrease in circulation to the brain due to hardening of the arteries.

Carotidnynia: A migraine-like syndrome characterized by tenderness, swelling, and occasional pulsation of the carotid artery in the neck. This condition is frequently misdiagnosed. Its treatment is like that of migraine.

Catecholamines: Biologically active substances related to adrenalin that have a marked effect on the nervous and cardiovascular systems. The metabolism of these may have some effect on migraine and has a definite effect on depression headaches.

CT scan: Computerized axial tomography produces thousands upon thousands of pictures. It utilizes X-rays which are combined by a computer into a single picture. This process enables the physician to make serial sections of the brain without invading the brain itself. It is used primarily to rule out organic disease as a cause of the headache problem. A CAT scan can be performed with or without dye. The dye may enhance the detection of a brain tumor or a blood clot.

Central sensitization: A condition in which the nervous system becomes regulated in a persistent state of high reactivity. Central sensitization is thought to play an integral role in the pain of migraine.

Cerebral aneurysm rupture: A condition caused by bleeding from a weakened or ballooned-out blood vessel. Most commonly it is hereditary. The headache resembles that associated with stroke and is of a very severe nature. Patients with an aneurysm rupture require immediate treatment. If the blood vessel blow-out is not complete or of only a minimal degree, surgery can sometimes treat this type of hemorrhage successfully.

Cerebral atrophy: A condition in which the brain deteriorates. It is usually diagnosed by MRI. The MRI will show marked enlargement of the brain ridges and the openings between them.

Cerebrospinal fluid: A clear, colorless liquid that cushions or protects the brain and spinal column. It increases or decreases in amount with the expansion or contraction of the brain. When the amount of spinal fluid is radically increased, it can cause headache. Usually, this increase is due to organic disease, but it can increase for no obvious reason.

Cervicogenic headache: Headache caused by a disorder of the cervical spine and its component bony disc and/or soft tissue elements, usually but not always accompanied by neck pain.

Chronic migraine: When migraine has transformed to the point that headaches occur on 15 or more days per month.

Chiari malformation: A condition in which brain tissue extends into the spinal canal. Most Chiari malformations are asymptomatic, but it is a potential cause of headache in patients. Only the most severe Chiari malformations are corrected with surgery.

Chronic paroxysmal hemicrania: A condition in which the patient gets multiple (15 to 20) headaches per day of short duration. It occurs more commonly in women. These patients are responsive to therapy with an anti-inflammatory drug such as indomethacin.

Chronic posttraumatic headache: Headache which develops within seven days of head injury and persists beyond three months.

Cluster headache: A one-sided headache usually occurring in or around one eye and typically of short duration, usually lasting several minutes to several hours at the most. It is called cluster because it occurs in a group or series. The patient has tearing of the eye, nasal congestion, facial flushing, and constriction of the pupil on the side of the headache. The series may last several months, occurring more frequently in the fall and spring, and the headaches may disappear for several months or several years. Some forms of cluster headache, however, occur chronically. Cluster headache occurs more commonly in males.

Cognitive behavioral therapy: A systematic approach of therapy that addresses dysfunctional emotions, behaviors, and thought processes through goal-oriented psychotherapy.

Complicated migraine: A type of migraine headache associated with neurological manifestations. Although rare, permanent damage to the brain and the retina may be caused by migraine. Frequently, distortions of the visual field, paralysis, and anesthesia occur as residuals of these migraine attacks.

Confusional states with migraine: It is not uncommon in young migraine sufferers to find confusion and disorientation as a presenting sign of the migraine attack. Prolonged stupors or comatose states have been associated with migraine, lasting up to seven days.

Depression: This emotional state may be one of the contributing factors in chronic migraine. It is often accompanied by a sleep disturbance in the form of frequent and early waking. Migraine patients with frequent attacks often have depression as one of the complications of their migraines. Also, patients with chronic pain syndromes are often markedly depressed.

Dihydroergotamine: An injectable form of ergotamine tartrate which is very helpful to cluster or migraine patients and does not have as many side effects as oral forms of ergotamine tartrate.

Divalproex Sodium (Depakote): Antiepileptic drug used to prevent seizures. This medication is also FDA-approved for migraine prevention.

Doppler Ophthalmic Test (DOT): A noninvasive test done with an instrument measuring blood flow to the superficial circulation of the eye. It determines if there is a decreased blood flow to the carotid arteries of the brain. This decrease may be significant since it may cause a small stroke and headache-like symptoms in older patients. Once diagnosed, strokes from this cause can be prevented.

341

Encephalitis: An inflammation of the brain itself, usually caused by a bacteria or virus, and serious cause of headache. The bacteria type can be treated with antibiotics. The viral type may cause continual headache after the infection has subsided, as well as permanent neurological problems.

Endorphins and enkephalins: The most common bodily-produced polypeptides. It has been determined that the brain produces these morphine-like substances to counteract painful syndromes.

Epilepsy: A condition in which seizures occur. Although causality has not been established, migraine appears to be more common among patients with epilepsy than among the general population.

Ergotamine: One of the drugs used to abort migraine. It is basically a vasoconstrictor, preventing the blood vessels from swelling. Since it does not decrease the cerebral blood pulse, it can be used for both classical and nonclassical migraine. The original drug comes from a mold that grows on rye, and the name is derived from the French word ergot. In the Middle Ages, eating bread made from moldy rye could be poisonous, causing gangrene of the hands and feet—a condition sometimes known as "St. Anthony's Fire." When the affected individuals went to St. Anthony's Shrine in Egypt, which was outside the infected area, they stopped eating the infected bread, and the malady was "miraculously" cured.

Estrogens: Estrogens are female hormones. If taken in the form of birth-control pills or postmenopausal treatment, they can increase the frequency, duration, severity, and complications of migraine.

Exertional headaches: With exercise, the muscles of the head, neck, and scalp require more blood, and this causes a swelling or vasodilation, which can cause head pain. Exertional headaches can, in some instances, be a sign of organic disease, and anyone that develops a severe headache following running, coughing, sneezing, bowel movement, or other exertions should certainly be checked to rule out any organic cause. The Diamond Headache Clinic has done extensive studies on both short- and long-lasting exertional headaches. It has been found that those that are benign and not due to organic disease are responsive to therapy with the drug indomethacin (Indocin).

Extracranial: Referring to things outside the skull, scalp, and the muscles that cover the head.

Facial pain: Chronic facial pain can be very confusing both to the patient and physician. It is most difficult to treat and is frequently unresponsive to therapy. Patients with facial pain are easily habituated or addicted to analgesic medications. It may be caused by migraine-like syndromes, muscular syndromes such as TMJ, herpetic or rheumatic disease, or it may be purely psychogenic.

Fiorinal: An analgesic medication made from aspirin, butalbital (a barbiturate), and caffeine with or without codeine phosphate for the treatment of tension headaches.

Gamma knife: Gamma knife is not actually a knife at all, but a device that concentrates cobalt radiation into a small space for the treatment of brain tumors. It was invented at the Karolinska Institute in Sweden in 1967.

Glaucoma: A group of eye diseases characterized by increased pressure within the eye, which can cause headache. With a sudden and acute obstruction, the pain can be severe and terrifying. With a gradual increase of eye pressure, the pain may be more moderate in nature. Intraocular pressure should be measured in headache patients. This procedure can be performed in any physician's office. Drugs used to treat depression may, in rare cases of glaucoma, cause an increase in intraocular pressure if the canal in which the eye fluids drain is inadequate.

Glossopharyngeal neuralgia: A rare inflammation of the ninth cranial nerve (the glossopharyngeal nerve). The pain is intermittent and severe, and is usually described as being around one side of the tonsillar area, the outer ear, the back of the tongue, or the angel of the jaw. The attacks can be induced by coughing, talking, or swallowing. Treatment is similar to that for trigeminal neuralgia or tic douloureux and is usually effective.

Greater occipital nerve: The nerve that supplies sensations to the scalp and back of the head. Because of its tortuous course between bone and muscle

343

substance, it is particularly vulnerable to trauma and pressure. Since this nerve supplies sensation to the major portion of the skull, pressure on it can cause a headache-like syndrome, sometimes called occipital neuralgia.

Head jolts: Certain headaches are particularly sensitive to head jolts because of swelling of the pain-sensitive blood vessels covering the brain. In this group are hangover headache, post-spinal puncture headache, post-concussion headache, or headache associated with meningitis or inflammation of the brain. A headache due to a brain tumor can also be sensitive to head jolts. Migraine or tension-type headache are usually not sensitive to jolting or position changes of the head.

Hemicrania continua: One-sided headache that is, by definition, responsive to treatment with indomethacin.

Hemiplegic migraine: A very rare form of migraine in which there is paralysis of the arm or leg on one side of the body. The paralysis can occur before, during, or after the onset of a headache. The attacks are usually temporary, but they may be prolonged and can rarely cause some permanent paralysis. In familial hemiplegic migraine, there is a family history of headaches with similar symptoms. Genetic mutations have been identified in familial hemiplegic migraine.

Histamine: A normal substance present in the body, which is released if tissues are injured. Histamine has been implicated as one of the substances in the blood considered to be a causative factor in cluster headache, and it has also been considered a provocative factor in migraine headaches. If histamine is given to a migraine patient, it can provoke a migraine-like headache. Histamine desensitization is a treatment used in chronic cluster headache.

Hormone therapy: Statements about hormonal supplemental therapy: 1. Older oral contraceptives which had a larger concentration of estrogen provoked more frequent migraines almost 80 percent of the time. Newer, lower-dose contraceptives which contain estrogen can still cause a problem at least one-third of the time. So, look for a change in headache pattern if you get put on them. 2. Cardio and cerebrovascular issues. Patients with migraine have a slight increased risk of stroke which is a little higher if you have migraine with aura. Adding estrogen to the mix further increases the risk as estrogen increases the risk of thromboembolic events. So, as women age it is generally consensus that over 35 years of age we caution to use a nonestrogen containing pill and that if you have migraine with aura a progestin-only pill may be better. 3. Patches and rings with estrogen confer the same risk. 4. Anyone who smokes should not take an estrogen-based product.

Horner's syndrome: Symptoms include drooping of the eyelid and constriction of the pupil with an injection to the white part of the eye, along with nasal congestion or drip. Some of these symptoms are also seen in cluster headache, or they can be a sign of severe neurological disease.

Hostility: Although not a primary cause, suppressed anger or repressed hostility can be a precipitant of migraine headaches. It is often but not always present in migraine-prone individuals.

Hot dog headache: A severe headache that usually starts within three-quarters of an hour after eating foods with sodium nitrite (used as a preservative in many meats, such as hot dogs, bacon, ham, and salami). It is added to prevent the bacteria of botulism and to give a uniform red color to the meat. Migraine sufferers are more prone to this type of headache.

Hypertension or high blood pressure: Hypertension is not a common cause of headache unless it is a malignant type, with a systolic pressure of over 180 mm Hg and a diastolic pressure of over 110 mm Hg. Most of the headache complaints of patients with milder hypertension are probably related to severe anxiety over their illness or other external factors. If the headache is due to severe hypertension, it is usually worse in the morning and decreases in intensity as the day continues.

Hypnic headache: A type of headache that begins during sleep and wakes the patient. Usually the headache lasts 15 minutes to 3 hours.

Hypnosis: A type of treatment in which the therapist puts the patient in a subconscious state. The objective manifestations of the mind become inactive, enabling the patient to relax and forget his head pain. Hypnosis has not been found to be an effective method of therapy for patients with cluster headache problems.

Hypoxia: A lack of oxygen which, coupled with an increase of carbon dioxide in the blood, has been observed to cause a swelling of the blood vessels of the brain. It is for this reason that some people get a headache at high altitudes. The headache often appears hours after exposure to low oxygen tension and is not relieved by the administration of oxygen. This factor has clinical significance because it has been theorized that low oxygen tension and hypoxia may be the initiating factor in all migraine attacks. A group of drugs, known as calcium antagonists, which will soon be available in the United States, act to prevent cerebral anoxia. These drugs may be effective in the prevention of migraine.

Ibuprofen: A nonsteroidal anti-inflammatory drug (NSAID) used as a pain reliever.

Ice cream headache: Ice cream lovers can experience intense, brief pain in the throat, head, or face after biting into ice cream or placing a spoonful against the back part of the roof of the mouth. The headache can occur when any cold substance is similarly positioned. The pain can be excruciating but disappears within a few minutes. Some investigators have reported that this type of headache occurs more frequently in people who are prone to migraine.

Idiopathic intracranial hypertension: Formerly known as pseudo tumor cerebri. A condition of increased intracranial pressure for which no specific cause is known. Usually, despite extensive laboratory testing, one cannot determine an obvious cause such as brain tumor, high blood pressure, and so forth. It may be due to menstrual dysfunction, hormone deficiency, hypothyroidism, or excessive intake of antibiotics or vitamin A. A prominent sign of this condition is marked congestion and distortion of the optic nerve as it enters the retina. The term "papilledema" is used to describe this state.

346

Inflammation: A response of the body to irritation or injury. For example, in an injury such as physical trauma with swelling, accompanying the swelling there is a rush of various blood cells into the affected areas, producing redness, swelling, and warmth.

Lower half migraine: A type of migraine in which the pain is felt in the face or around the ear or even as low as the cheeks or jaw; or it may have a distribution like that found in cluster headache. The pain is often less severe, less sharp, and may last longer than regular migraine attacks. It is difficult to treat.

Medication overuse headache (MOH): Headache which occurs on 15 or more days per month in a patient overusing one or more medications for more than three months. For opioids, combination analgesics (such as Excedrin), and triptans overuse is defined as greater than10 doses per month. For NSAIDs and simple analgesics, overuse is 15 or more days per month for more than three months.

Meningitis: An inflammation of the brain coverings that is almost always associated with headache. The inflammation causes a stiff neck, which is typical of meningitis, and a high temperature. Immediate care is necessary. A spinal tap will usually confirm the diagnosis of meningitis and with modern antibiotics, about 99 percent of the cases can be cured. The headache is not chronic, but acute.

Menstrual migraine: Migraine that occurs *exclusively* with a woman's menstrual period. A drop in estrogen levels during these times may be a precipitating cause. Menstrual migraine can be adequately treated with triptans or anti-inflammatory drugs prior to and during a woman's period.

Menstrual-related migraine: Migraine that occurs prior to or during the menstrual period, in a woman who also gets migraines at other times.

Migraine equivalents: A term for migraine that exhibits itself in forms other than head pain. A diagnosis of migraine equivalent is determined by a previous history of typical migraine attacks, no evidence of organic lesions, and the replacement of normal headaches by an equivalent group of symptoms. It is

347

important in these cases to determine the presence of a family history of migraine. Also, it is characteristic that drugs used to treat migraine will help the equivalent symptom. The most frequent migraine equivalent is "abdominal migraine," which is characterized by recurrent episodes of vomiting and abdominal pain without the symptom of headache. The bouts of pain can last anywhere from one to seven hours. Abdominal migraine occurs more frequently in female children. Patients characteristically show yawning, listlessness, and drowsiness during their attacks. Many people with abdominal migraine have undergone unnecessary abdominal surgery. A migraine equivalent may also be characterized by visual symptoms such as blind spots, seeing half the field of vision, or loss of vision without the migraine headache. Another type of equivalent is psychic migraine, in which the patient exhibits transient mood disorders or erratic behavior as part of or in place of the headache syndrome.

Migraine with aura: Formerly known as classic migraine. Differentiated from migraine without aura by the occurrence of a warning or aura prior to the acute attack. Many neurologists classify any migraine attack in which there are neurological manifestations as classical migraine. A migraine patient usually also has the following symptoms: nausea, or sick vomiting, a one-sided headache, and a family history of headache.

Migraine without aura: Migraine exhibiting one-sidedness, nausea, vomiting, photophobia, and hereditary history. The aura or prodrome is absent.

Mindfulness: A process of focusing on slow, diaphragmatic breathing and putting oneself in the "moment."

MRA: Magnetic resonance angiography uses MRI (magnetic resonance imaging) technology to record images of blood vessels to find stenosis, occlusions, and other abnormalities.

MRI: Magnetic resonance imaging uses a magnetic field and radio wave energy to create images of the body's internal structures. It presents a different set of information than X-rays or computed tomography (CT) scans.

MSG (monosodium glutamate) headache: It has been found that monosodium glutamate can cause headaches or other symptoms in susceptible people. It is often added to Chinese foods, with wonton soup a frequent offender. However, it is also found in many processed meats and tenderizers. Symptoms occur within 30 minutes of ingesting MSG, as it is rapidly absorbed by the stomach. Although the headache chiefly affects the temples, there may also be perspiration, tightness, and pressure over the face and chest. (*See also Asian restaurant syndrome.*)

New Daily Persistent Headache (NDPH): The rapid development (within three days) of an unrelenting headache in a person with very little or no headache history. NDPH does not evolve from episodic migraine or episodic tension-type headache but is a new headache.

Nicotine: The nicotine found in cigarettes and other smoking materials can increase the frequency and duration of migraine attacks. Excessive smoking can also be a factor in cluster headache attacks.

Nitrates and nitrites: Nitrates are used to treat coronary heart disease and nitrites are used as food additives to prevent botulism in meats. Both substances can increase vasodilation and thus increase the tendency toward migraine attacks.

OnabotulinumtoxinA (BOTOX): A neurotoxin developed to treat a variety of conditions by relaxing muscles through decreasing nerve signals to muscles. It is FDA-approved for the prevention of chronic migraine and is administered with injections every three months.

Ophthalmoplegic migraine: A rare type of headache that occurs in children or young adults. Associated with the headache, there is paralysis of the third nerve and there may be drooping of the eyelid, dilation of the pupils, and paralysis of the eye muscles. This is a temporary type of migraine, and patients usually have a family history of similar attacks.

349

Oral contraceptives: The estrogen in oral contraceptives and in postmenopausal hormones may increase the frequency, duration, severity, and complications of migraine.

Papilledema: A condition that occurs following an inflammation of the optic nerve at the point of entrance into the eyeball. On examination, inflammation or swelling of the optic nerve can be observed. It is usually caused by increased intracranial pressure but can be caused by a brain tumor pressing on the optic nerve. It is an excellent indicator for the physician seeking to determine an organic cause of headache.

Pheochromocytoma: A tumor of the adrenal gland which causes marked transient elevations of blood pressure and may provoke symptoms that mimic migraine disease. A simple blood or urine test can differentiate migraine from this disorder.

Placebo: A drug or treatment that has no medical benefit but whose success is related to the suggestion that it will work. Thus, placebo response refers to the beneficial effect that a placebo medication will have when given to certain individuals. It is estimated that about 25 to 30 percent of individuals will have a placebo response to drugs.

Platelet antagonists: A group of drugs containing a substance that prevents the platelets from disintegrating or clumping together. These drugs may have significance in the treatment of migraine since the platelets contain the chemical serotonin, implicated as one of the causes of migraine.

Polymyalgia rheumatica: A medical condition which usually occurs after age 55 in which there are marked muscular and rheumatic pains. Temporal arteritis, which can cause a severe form of headache as well as blindness, is one manifestation of polymyalgia rheumatica. It is essential to identify this condition for proper treatment.

Polypeptides: Amino acids which may have some pain and headache prevention qualities, but may also cause headaches. They are normally present in the brain. The ones being investigated currently are the endorphins and enkephalins, which are morphine-like substances.

Pregnancy: Migraine will usually disappear by the end of second month of pregnancy, only to reappear after the delivery of the baby. Migraine rarely occurs from the end of the second month of pregnancy to birth because of hormonal changes.

Prodrome: Symptoms that may occur before a migraine attack. They may take the form of a feeling of elation, a clearer awareness of color, variations in moods, an increase in energy, or a feeling of hunger or thirst. Conversely, some patients may get a feeling of depression.

Prolactin: A hormone released by the pituitary gland. There has been an increase in the number of cases of benign tumors of the pituitary gland with headache as one of the symptoms. It most often occurs in young adults. This hormone can be easily measured in the blood and, if markedly elevated, more sophisticated pituitary tests can be performed. An increase in prolactin is usually accompanied by an increase in breast size, discharge from the breasts, or irregular periods.

Prostacyclin: A substance similar to prostaglandin which is released by the wall of a blood vessel and has the opposite effect of prostaglandin. It prevents the platelets from aggregating or clumping together and may cause the blood vessels to dilate; therefore having a prophylactic effect on migraine headaches.

Prostaglandins: A group of approximately 14 chemical substances released by various organs. The first one identified was released by the prostate, thereby earning the name "prostaglandins." One prostaglandin in particular may provoke migraine by causing the platelets to aggregate or clump together, thereby causing a release of serotonin. These substances also have a marked effect on the blood vessels and smooth muscles and are part of an inflammatory reaction. Thus, prostaglandin release can be a causative factor in headache, and substances that negate the action of prostaglandins can help decrease the frequency, severity, and duration of headache.

351

Pseudotumor cerebri: *See idiopathic intracranial hypertension.*

Ptosis: Drooping of the eyelid, usually on one side of the head. It can be a sign of organic disease but most commonly is a symptom of cluster headache.

Raeder's syndrome: A syndrome similar to cluster headache and usually treated in the same way. Some practitioners would like to consider it a separate condition.

Rebound headache: *See medication overuse headache.*

St. Anthony's Fire: A syndrome from the Middle Ages in which fever, redness, gangrene, and other symptoms appeared after the eating of bread made from moldy flour on which ergotamine had formed.

Scotoma: A blind spot of varying size which may occur within the field of vision. Scotomas are sometimes present with the onset of migraine headaches as part of the aura.

Sella turcica: The cavity in the brain that encases the pituitary gland. When the cavity is enlarged or somewhat distorted, it can signify the presence of a brain tumor.

Serotonin: A chemical substance primarily present in the central nervous system, gastrointestinal (GI) tract, and platelets. It is a neurotransmitter, meaning it is involved in the transmission of signals between nerves. Serotonin has an impact on mood, and it is thought to be involved in the mechanism of migraine.

Sinusitis: The area affected by sinus headache is usually above the eyes (frontal sinus) or below the eyes (maxillary sinus). Headache very often follows an upper respiratory infection which blocks the sinuses. The pain is caused by a stretching of the lining of these open cavities and the formation of pus within the sinuses, which will not drain. Often, the areas above or below the eyes where the sinuses are located, are very tender. Chronic sinus disease rarely causes head pain. Acute sinusitis, associated with a fever and a blocked sinus, can cause acute head pain. One of the most commonly seen misdiagnosis of headache is when migraine is misdiagnosed as sinus headache.

Skin or allergy testing: Not relevant in migraine diagnosis or therapy. Allergy desensitization is not helpful in migraine treatment.

Strokes: It is true that migraine patients are at a slight increased risk of stroke, and, yes certain strokes can produce headache as an initial symptom. Patients with a cerebral hemorrhage almost always have a headache, particularly as the blood enters the spinal fluid. However, this is only a transient type of headache and the stroke symptoms, such as paralysis, are the ones that predominate. Of note, migraine patients who experience aura are at a further increased risk of stroke over those without aura.

Temporal arteritis: A vascular disease characterized by inflammation of blood vessels, which produces a very severe headache and usually strikes people over age 55. The arteries in the temple are thicker and more tortuous than normal vessels. In some cases, patients may have other bodily symptoms such as loss of appetite, or joint and muscle pain. A simple sedimentation rate or C-reactive protein (blood tests) will suggest this diagnosis because it if often quite elevated. A biopsy of the temporal artery, which lies just below the skin, confirms the diagnosis. It is important that the patient receive immediate treatment because the condition can lead to blindness.

Temporomandibular joint dysfunction (TMJ): This diagnosis is probably one of the most overused terms relating to head pain. Symptoms include localized facial pain, limited jaw movements, muscle tenderness, and sensations when moving the jaw up and down. Usually, X-rays of this joint are normal. The pain is most often described as being located in front, behind the ear on the affected side, and may radiate over the cheeks and face. Some people will complain of a sensation of blockage in the ear. Thousands of dollars have been spent on unnecessary procedures. The treatment is focused on relief of the muscle spasms by using simple tranquilizers or muscle relaxants. Moist heat massage is also helpful. However, dental splints are rarely helpful. Patients must be cautioned against extensive reconstructions of the mouth, since they are usually not indicated or useful.

Tension-type headache: Formerly called muscle contraction headache. A nonspecific headache, which is not vascular or migrainous, and is not related to organic disease. It is caused by a tightening of the muscles at the back of the neck and of the face and scalp. Muscle contraction headache is a steady, mild headache, and is sometimes described as having a band-like or hat-band distribution around the head. It can occur episodically, that is, occasionally, or once or twice a month, and is usually best treated with simple aspirin or acetaminophen (Tylenol) compounds. The simple, episodic tension headache is often associated with fatigue and the stresses of life. These people rarely consult a physician for their headaches. Those who do seek help from a physician often have chronic tension-type headache.

Third ventricle cyst: A rare, nonmalignant type of growth that blocks the spinal fluid from flowing on its normal route from the ventricles into the spinal cord. There is a narrow passage in the middle of the brain, where a cyst may prevent the normal flow of the fluid. The typical headache characteristic of this condition will occur during changes of position. Surgery is usually required.

Tic douloureux (trigeminal neuralgia): Episodes of severe shooting or stabbing pain on one side of the face which are generated by eating, talking, shaving, or cold drafts. The painful spasms last a few seconds and are severe and intolerable. Tic douloureux most commonly occurs after the age of 50 and is more frequent in women. It can be treated medically or surgically.

Topiramate: Antiepileptic drug used in the prevention of seizures. This medication is also FDA-approved for migraine prevention.

Transcutaneous electrical neurostimulation: The use of electrical currents to alleviate headache pain. It has been used extensively in treating cluster and migraine headaches but has not proved to be an effective form of therapy.

Trigeminal neuralgia: *See Tic douloureux.*

Triptans: A group of tryptamine-based medications used in the treatment of migraine and cluster headaches.

Tumor: The greatest fear of all headache patients is that their headache is caused by a brain tumor. However, this is uncommon; only one-tenth of one percent of all headache patients suffer from a brain tumor. Their history consists of a recent onset of headache with increasing severity. The headache is made worse by exertion such as coughing, sneezing, or running, and the patient may exhibit some other neurological symptoms such as changes in handwriting, personality, and thought. Upon examination by a physician, there may be some defect in either motor, sensory, or brain reflex activity.

Tyramine: A naturally occurring substance in the protein of the body, which is also found in certain foods and beverages. Ingestion of these foods can cause more frequent migraine attacks.

Vasoconstriction: A narrowing or a clamping down of the blood vessel.

Vasodilatation: A swelling or distention of a blood vessel.

Vasomotor rhinitis: A congestion of the nose, which can be triggered by a variety of stimuli such as temperature change, exercise, change of position, humidity, and odors. It is rarely an allergic reaction. A patient may exhibit a mild headache with vasomotor-rhinitis-like symptoms.

Weather-related headache: Studies conducted by a Swedish research group have recorded headache attacks in relation to climatic factors such as atmospheric pressure, outdoor temperature, wind velocity, cloudiness, relative humidity, and precipitation. An increased headache frequency was associated with high temperature, low pressure, and high wind velocity. It was concluded that climatic factors influence headache frequency.

Made in the USA
San Bernardino, CA
01 November 2018